5.0

# Tennis Secrets

By Richard Hasse.

In collaboration with the

Tennis Think Tank.

All rights reserved. No part of this book may be reproduced in any form or by any means without permission in writing from the author.

First Edition

A large portion of the profits from this book are used to provide rackets to young intercity tennis players.

Dedicated to Maggie

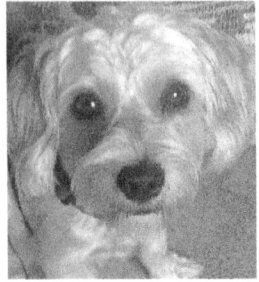

A fun loving doggie who never takes her eye off the ball.


And to Marvin Dent

You're correct Marvin. Federer is Betterer.

# Table of Contents

Forward ---------------------------------------------------------------- 4
The Stroke ------------------------------------------------------------- 8
Rethink Open, Closed, and Neutral Racket Face ---------------- 12
The Sweet Area ------------------------------------------------------ 15
Visualizing Impact Configurations ------------------------------- 17
The Spot Target ~ a Simple Effective Targeting System ----- 32
Hold Your Focus on the Impact Point --------------------------- 38
The Most Important Tool That a Player Has ------------------- 39
Make the Magic ------------------------------------------------------ 42
Tennis Cybernetics ------------------------------------------------- 48
The Tennis Concentration Trance ------------------------------- 56
The End All, Be All of Strategy ---------------------------------- 61
The Four Response Modes ---------------------------------------- 65
The Average Approach to Tennis -------------------------------- 72
The Champion's Pattern ------------------------------------------- 76
When Coaches Blame Their Athletes --------------------------- 91
Move Your Center Of Mass into the Impact Point ------------ 93
Linear and Rotational Momentum on the Ball ----------------- 95
Roll the Spot Target ------------------------------------------------ 100
How to Prepare for a Match -------------------------------------- 101
Understand the Continental Grip -------------------------------- 128
Footwork Goals ------------------------------------------------------ 130
Conclusion ------------------------------------------------------------ 134

# Forward

A player's eyesight is the most important tool that they have. Few players understand how their eyesight works on a physical, mechanical, anatomical level. Roger Federer has the greatest achievement record of all time because he uses an identical or similar system to the one outlined in this book. He may be doing this by plan or it may come natural to him. An understanding of the exact mental state for tennis also needs to be looked at. This book presents an organized approach to the game that a tennis player can use when the ball is up.

Stroke production skills are not presented in a conventional manner. Tennis has approached "hull speed" in terms of the bio-mechanical efficiently of each shot. It is the one aspect that we are best at. Stroke production skills are best learned on court from a talented pro or coach. Your strokes will always be the foundation of your game. The approach presented in this book will improve your strokes as a bi-product of better visual skills and better practice habits. Of course, you need to learn to hit the ball correctly. This book concentrates on what you need to do once you know how to hit the ball.

There are six variables about each impact. Some are important for placement and some are important for error elimination. It is easier to understand one variable if you understand all of them. The strategy system is a simple pattern that most pros use. It is impossible to use this, "Champion's Pattern" if you cannot hit the ball to a specific small area of the court. The strategy is impossible without placement. The "Magic Number" is an evaluation tool used to gage any tennis workout or cooperative practice session. Make sure you understand this concept. Just like any other sport, tennis matches are won and lost not only on game day but, also in practice and training. That is why much of this book is devoted to practice, training, and preparation.

The spot target and the tip target are two very valuable skills that can help any player at any level. However, this book was written with a mature, strong, experienced player in mind. If you want to improve your game one or two NTRP levels or even play at the highest levels then this book is for you.

We wish to thank the following pros for their scorching and impassioned feedback of the original version. Without their input, this book would have been a horrible read and not much help:

Ken Cussick Jr., Mike Baugh, Jeremy Reynolds, Eric Dobsha, Roy Coopersmith, Jon Wharton, Greg Lumb, Matthew Austin Mathes, Seth Aaron Hoffman, Don Petrine, Aviram Markovich, David Contois, Michael Paduch, Roberto M. Ancira, Jeremy Kokry, Patrick Horne, Bill Patton, Styrling Strothe, & Lucile Bosche. I hope that I have not left anyone out. We are forever in your debt.

The Tennis Think Tank

A formal think tank is a group of individuals who use a communication, reflection, and revisiting technique to find a method, a solution, or a new approach to a problem. A group of five individuals contacted me after reading my first book, <u>Thirty Things all Great Tennis Players Know</u>. They felt that I had a good book but it could be improved upon. They wanted a shorter book that focused less on technique. These five individuals do not wish to be acknowledged. One of them is an optometrist, two are former NCAA coaches, all are 5.0 or above players. I am a former high school coach, private instructor and have been a part of many instructional teams at camps, clinics, junior development groups, and team formats. I have multiple Open and 5.0 tournament first place victories in singles, doubles and mixed doubles. I have also been the primary practice partner to 3 Texas State High School singles champions and one U.S. Open participant. I am a lifelong player and student of the game.

This book was think tanked using the following method:

Every decision was made by each member commenting in an online chat. Each person would give their thoughts until all had nothing more to add. Then we would wait 48 hours and consider what had been communicated by each person. This reflective period is the key to a think tank's success.


After 48 hours we would have another online chat and reach a decision. This is how we decided what needed to be added, changed, re-worded, or eliminated.

After the original version was complete we waited another 48 hours and then asked several teaching pros to review the book. We used several online coaching forums to do this. All of the pros mentioned in the Forward reviewed the first draft. The pros were very open, honest, and pulled no punches. The most valuable feedback came from pros who disagreed with our approach. This feedback usually pointed out where we were unclear or misunderstood. Each and every criticism was discussed, reflected on for 48 hours and then discussed again.

The Tennis Think Tank wishes to express our sincere appreciation for their time and thoughts. Only professionals who truly care about improving tennis would take their own time to review another group's book. Once again, we are forever in your debt.

The Tennis Think Tank thanks you for reading.

Chapter 1

# The Stroke

The stroking technique is important. The stroking technique is the second most important thing that you must practice. It is not the most important aspect of the game to concentrate on when a point is in progress. The stroking technique needs to be almost automatic when a point is in progress. In today's fast paced game, you have limited time to devote to the exact choreographed stroking form. Over emphasis on the exact technique of each shot is an ideal way to produce above average players. It is a great way to teach beginners and children. It does not produce world class or 5.0 singles players. There is a bottleneck at the 4.0-4.5 level. Many players reach the 4.0-4.5 level and then spend years or their entire tennis career never improving past this point. The over emphasis on what a stroke looks like does not work at the highest levels of the game. This approach worked in the 1980s. It will never work again. Your goal should be to reach at least the 5.0 level. 5.0 is like a black belt in tennis.

Your visual and mental skills are 50% of what you need to be successful at any level. This is the biggest secret to great tennis and the biggest thing that 5.0 players know. Racket-eye coordination and knowing how to hit the ball to a certain spot make up the most important half of the game. Where the ball lands is as important as what the stroke looks like. The good news is that these skills can be developed.

Almost the entire tennis world believes that stroke production skills are all that you need to play great tennis. Change this misconception or you will continue to be above average and below great, even if you have perfect looking strokes.

The goal of this book is to provide you with a blueprint that you can use to build a great game. Stoke production skills are the foundation of that game. This approach will build a great game on that foundation.

In a recent post, one well respected tennis writer named Marvin Dent, who talked with Federer, claims that Fed could not even tell you what kind of grips he used. Marvin claimed that Federer wore the racket, "like a glove with no fingers". It is obvious that Fed is less concerned with a strict technique than are those who study him. We cannot copy Federer's success by copying his strokes. His real skills are mental and visual. He visualizes the racket as an extension of his hand and targets each ball with strict visual discipline. The most common feedback received from several of the well-respected teaching pros and coaches who reviewed early versions of this book was the idea that the best players in the world could not describe how they hit the ball. In other words, they are concentrating on something else. They have gone beyond how to hit the ball and are using their mental resources for targeting and strategic play. Here is your world class technique:

1. Use the, "wear the racket like a glove with no fingers" analogy, or any other analogy that works for you. The important thing is that you visualize the racket as an extension of your hand.

2. Follow each incoming ball all the way to the string bed.

3. Catch the ball at a pre-planned spot on the string bed.

4. Keep your head down and your eyes focused on the impact point until the follow thru is complete.

This does not mean that what you know about stroke production is unimportant. It means that you cannot waste too much of your information processing resources on technique when the ball is up. Get your racket back, focus on the impact, follow through and recover. Stroke production is the one thing that most players have right. Many details are essential for success in tennis. The entire game of tennis is a game of habits. You must ritualize all important things as familiar habits. You will resort to the familiar when you are under pressure. There are about 30 critical skills that each player must master. Leaving any of the 30 or so things out will build a weakness into your game. Your visual skills are the glue that binds the rest of your game together.

If you master the visual skills presented in this book your strokes will improve as a byproduct of superior control and confidence.

The 5.0 player should be willing to play their best against any level opponent. The 5.0 player must master visual, strategic, physical, mental, and stroke production skills.

Your game should improve very quickly if are not ignoring these aspects of development.

Chapter 2

# Rethink Open, Closed, and Neutral Racket Face

Neutral Racket Face Angles:

Rethink a neutral racket face. The angle between the court and the racket face is irrelevant for a spin-less shot.

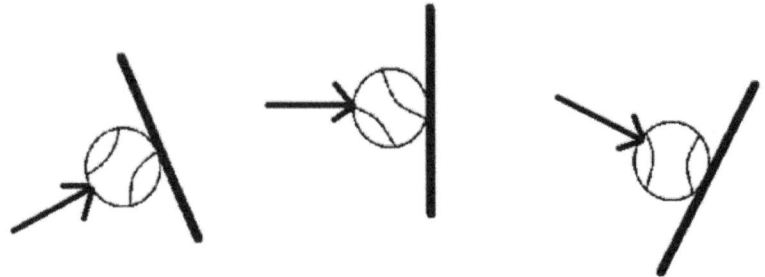

Neutral racket face angles relative to the trajectory at impact are often used to counter punch.

The angle between the trajectory of the incoming ball and the face of the racket is much more relevant than the angle between the racket face and the court surface. A trajectory has a changing flight line. Your highest percentage shot is to exactly reverse the path of the ball. Players who hit the ball on the middle two strings with the string bed perpendicular to the flight line of the ball have optimum control when they hit a shot without spin. This is a neutral face racket angle. This configuration will self-stabilize if the racket face moves exactly into the new trajectory and stays 90 degrees to the new trajectory. If you are taking the ball on the rise you must open the racket face slightly as the strings stretch.

This racket face is neutral to the flilght line. It is not an open face.

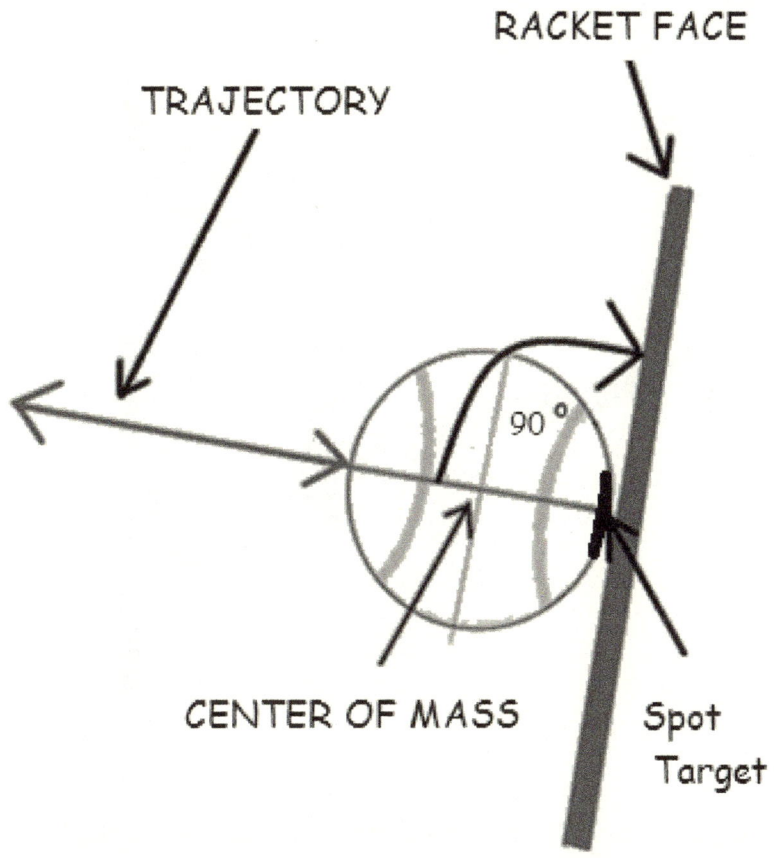

The angle is relative to the flight line not the court surface.

This picture is the impact configuration for a windshield wiper forehand.

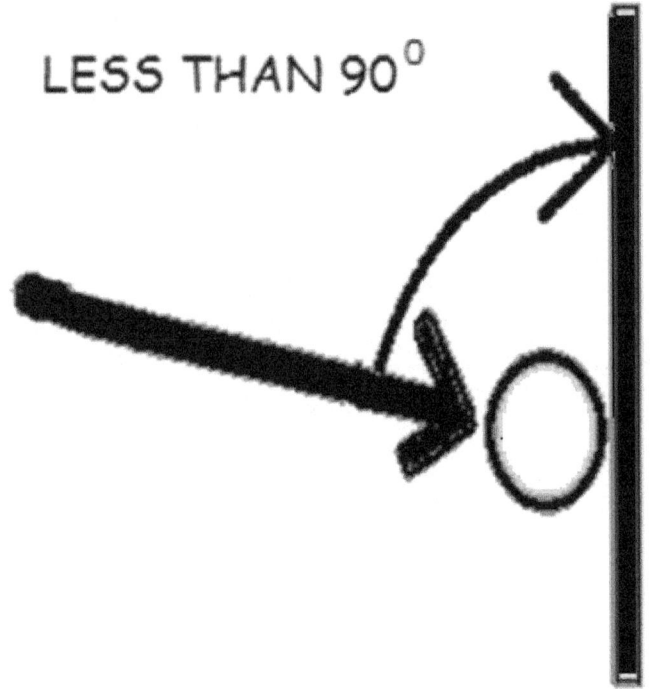

It is somewhat of an exception because it is usually 90 degrees to the court surface. The picture shows a closed face relative to the incoming flight line. The face of the racket will close further as the shot progresses.

Chapter 3

# The Sweet Area

There is a general state of denial about where on the string bed the ball should be taken. One teaching pro after another will tell you to take the ball on the two "main strings". Racket companies tell you about how good their racket is at resisting the tendency to twist on off center hits. But if you do any internet image or slow-motion video search of modern pros you will see that very few of them ever create spin by impacting the ball on the two "main strings". Today's rackets do not have a sweet spot. They have a sweet area. This huge sweet area is made even larger by modern multifilament strings. World class players typically use the outside edges of the sweet area because this will put more of the racket's mass above, below, or to the side of the ball. This will naturally cause the racket to roll over, under, or around the ball.

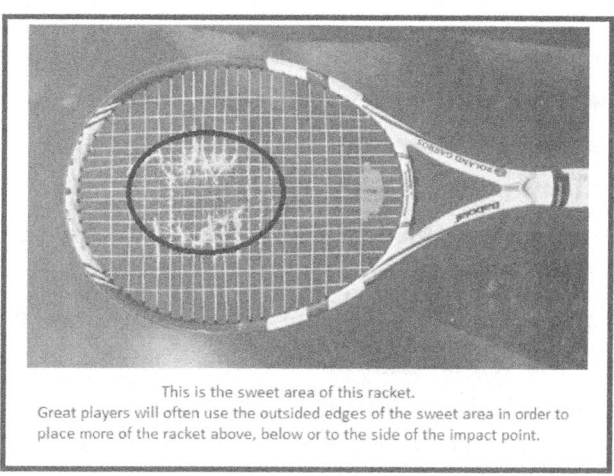

This is the sweet area of this racket.
Great players will often use the outsided edges of the sweet area in order to place more of the racket above, below or to the side of the impact point.

The sweet area is huge compared to rackets 50 years ago.

The monster size sweet area defines modern technique. The greatest players in the world are using the torque generated by an off center hit to their advantage on every spin shot that they hit. They do this by moving the impact point towards the trailing edge of the sweet area. Great topspin shots are taken below the hand and/or below the two main strings. Great slice shots are taken above the hand and/or above the two main strings. Only spin less shots are taken on the two main strings and level with the hand. Many great players will keep the impact in the center of the sweet area and raise, lower, or slant the racket tip so that the hand is above the ball during a topspin producing impact, below the ball for an under spin producing impact and slightly off the side when hitting a spin serve. It is actually very easy to catch the ball at an exact spot on the string bed if you are observing the impact.

Teaching pros and good players who consistently take the ball low on the string bed often claim that every shot should be hit on the two main strings. They are not following their own advice and they don't even know it, because: they are blind to the instant of impact. Most players at all levels are blind to the moment of impact. This is one of the main obstacles to becoming a great player. There is no understanding of the importance of visual and mental discipline. There is no understanding of the importance of impact configurations as they relate to spin and power. There is just BFMI.

Chapter 4

## Visualizing Impact Configurations

Here are diagrams of the acceptable impact configurations for topspin groundstrokes, under spin groundstrokes, and spin serves:

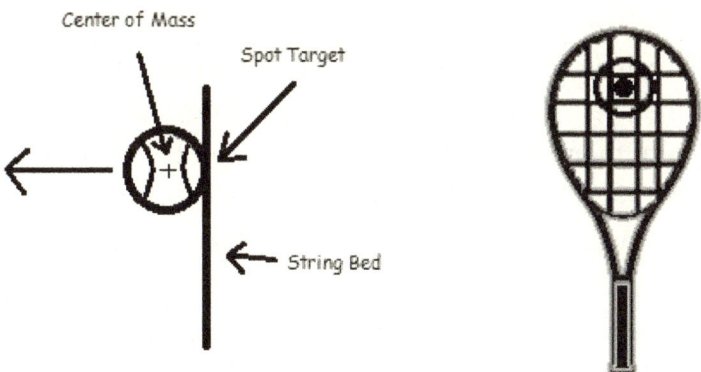

### Pronated Topspin Serve

Of course, all pronated serves begin with the racket moving as if you were trying to hit the ball with the frame instead of the strings. The pronation delivers more power at impact. You should jump into every serve.

The pronated straight topspin serve is impacted with the plane of the string bed at 90 degrees to the intended trajectory. The upper edge of the sweet area is the best impact point and will add velocity to the shot. The pronation snaps into this configuration at impact. Both the long and the cross strings should be at 90 degrees to the trajectory. Visualize a level trajectory. Topspin is created by driving the tip down at impact while keeping the elbow as high as possible.

You should visualize a straight line between the racket tip and the elbow. The pronated serve uses less wrist motion. You pronate with the elbow. This serve creates the power by using a straighter arm from the elbow. By keeping the elbow high during the impact, keeping the tip and the elbow more or less on a straight line, and driving the racket tip down; the power provided by the wrist is replace by power provided by the shoulder.

If you do not have a pronated serve to use as first strike weapon then you must do what it takes to develop one. If you get it right then it will be obvious. You will be hitting faster serves with less effort. If you do not see the results after trying to develop a pronated serve on your own the go to an experienced pro with a reputation for developing great players and drop the big bucks on lessons until you have this weapon. It is a must at the 5.0+ level.

## The Slice Serve

This serve uses more wrist than the pronated topspin serve. The racket snaps into this configuration at impact. Smash the spot target straight through the center of mass. At impact, you should favor the trailing edge of the sweet area and roll the spot target to three o'clock as the strings stretch. The linear vector for all serves is level with the court. Visualize this vector and add the rotation. Force the tip down as you are crushing the ball using as much wrist as possible. The follow thru should be tip down – butt plate up. This is much more important than what happens before the impact.

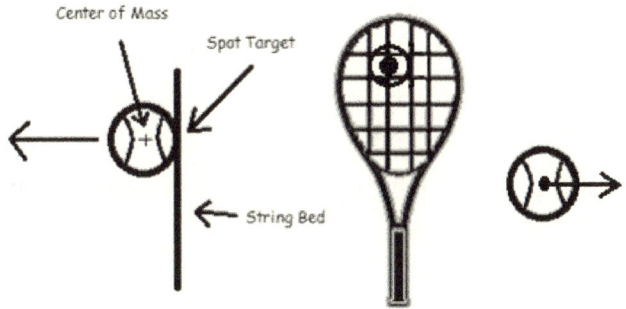

It takes raw applied strength, timing, reach and visual focus on the ball to hit a great serve. Apply all of your forearm and wrist strength at impact to drive the tip down. The hand should be well to the left of the ball as the power stroke begins. This configuration will place the hand just to the right of the ball at impact, not right under it. The hand should continue to move to the right and towards the net as the shot progresses. Visualize both vectors, Linear and Rotational!

Kick Serve

The kick serve is very similar to the slice serve. The stroke should look the same until impact. The racket snaps into this configuration at impact. You should make contact just before your racket is straight up. At impact, you should favor the trailing edge of the sweet spot area and roll the spot target to 1:30 or 2 o'clock. The linear vector is about the same for all serves. Crush the spot target level with the court as you are applying the rotational force.

The hand should be well to the left of the ball as the power stroke begins. The hand should be to the right of the ball at impact and moving to the right and up. Finish the impact for the kick serve by driving the tip down with all of your wrist strength as you are crushing the ball. The follow thru for all serves should be tip down – butt plate up.

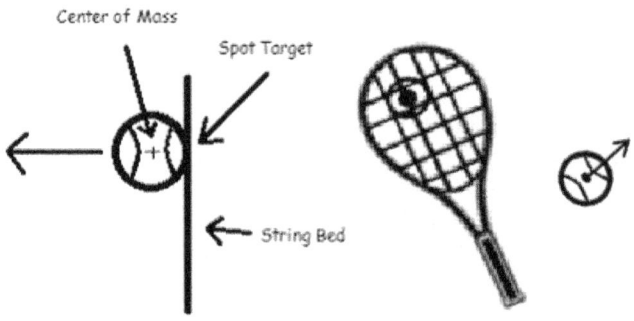

You must apply a linear force and a rotational force at the same time to produce an effective spin shot. Visualize both forces.

You have got to have a great serve to play 5.0+ tennis. Learn and practice all three serve until they are feared weapons. I have been around a ton of great players. The greatest players never neglect service practice.

## Spin-less Ground Stroke

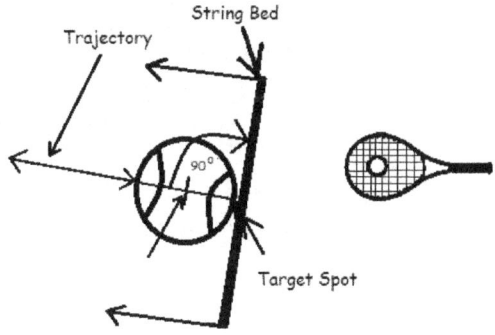

Crush the spot target through the center of mass keeping the racket face perpendicular to the trajectory. This shot will self-stabilize. The linear vector must be above level because you will not be providing lift when you roll the spot target. It is easiest to catch the ball as it is starting to descend. Once you begin to line up a spin less shot perpendicular to the descending trajectory you should be able to really hit a powerful fast spin-less shot. There is only one applied force at impact and one vector created. Visualize the first 4 inches or first two feet of the new trajectory line. An eastern or continental grip is used for this configuration.

This is a very effective counter punch and is an excellent shot to mix in with topspin and slice.

Slice Groundstrokes

For an under-spin shot it is best to visualize the outgoing trajectory about 8 degrees above level. This is the linear vector. If you do not visualize the outgoing trajectory you will put too many shots into the net. The racket will naturally roll under the ball. Roll the spot target down as you are creating the linear momentum. The hand should be well above the impact point at the beginning of the power stroke. The hand must be under the impact point when you are crushing and rolling the ball for the racket to help roll the spot target down.

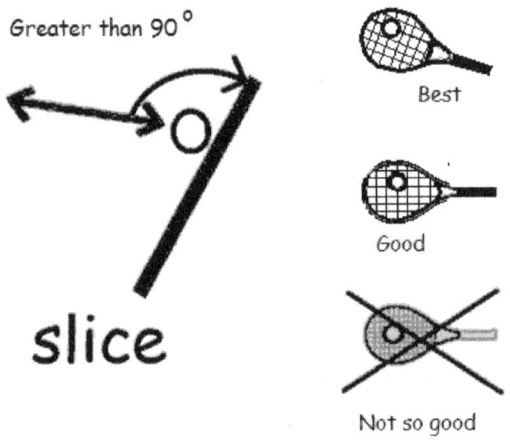

Most players use one of these two acceptable impact configurations for under-spin. Practice under-spin with the tip level with the handle and with the tip above the handle. Both of these configurations can be used with a slow too fast motion to throw the racket through the ball with massive power and spin.

Some will use both configurations to create shots that are similar but not exactly the same. Using both will confuse some opponents.

For maximum under spin drop the handle and impact the ball above the two middle long strings. This is the preferred configuration for crosscourt in the 50 - 50 zone.

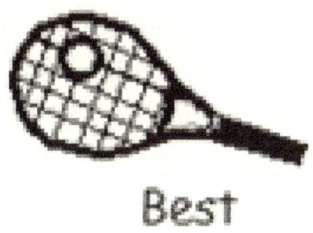

Best

This is a configuration that makes the slice a monster shot if it is taken above the shoulders.

For max power without sacrificing too much spin use a level racket and impact the ball above the two middle long strings just a little further from the tip.

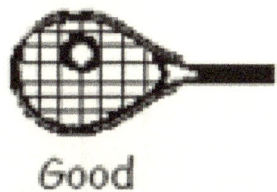

Good

Both can be used to create world class shots. Impacting the ball with the two middle long strings is seldom used to create a world class one-handed slice. Figure out what works for you. Use a continental grip and a slow too fast motion.

## Windshield Wiper Forehands

Topspin works best if you visualize the component vectors instead of the outgoing trajectory. Visualize a flat shot and the straight line in the direction that you want to hit to. Adjust the linear vector slightly up or down to perfect your depth and placement. The linear vector for all topspin shots should be level or slightly above level. Roll the spot target up using as much wrist as possible while the strings are stretched. The hand should be well below the intended impact point as the power stroke starts. The hand should be above the ball at impact. This will create a normal full power stroke. The parabolic trajectory will clear the net and dive down onto the court. This should be a monster shot. Learn to apply all of the linear and rotational force that you are able to control. The racket will roll over the ball. This is a diagram of what you visualize.

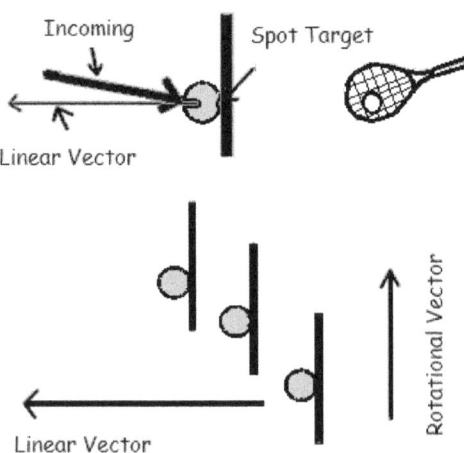

Never open up a racket face relative to the incoming trajectory if hitting with topspin. If the ball is going long it is because you are a beast and need to close the face a little more relative to the incoming trajectory. You must drop the racket head and get the hand above the impact point.

Dropping the tip and favoring the trailing edge of the sweet area will make it easier to impart spin to the ball. Use a semi-western grip with a racket that has the tip below the handle. This is an awesome shot that needs to be used as an attack weapon. This is the shot that defeats the grinding all court player.

Eastern Topspin

For awesome, accurate, consistent, and powerful topspin use a string bed with the long strings level and take the ball below the two middle long strings. Use an eastern grip with a level racket. The hand should be below the impact point at the beginning of the power stroke. The hand should be above the ball at impact. This is the workhorse, counter-punching, powerful ground stroke that is very easy to control. The racket face will roll over the ball and help create topspin.

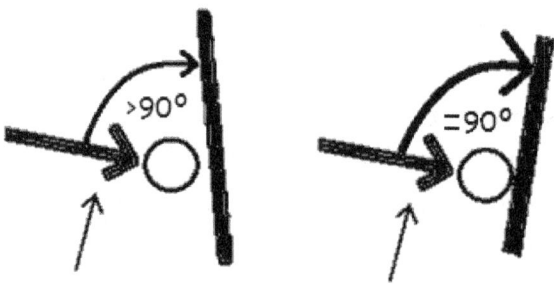

An Eastern Topspin Forehand can be hit with the string bed at 90 degrees or less relative to the incoming trajectory.

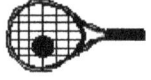

The configuration has the added benefit of being able to keep your opponent guessing. You can use the same grip and hit a spin less shot by taking the ball on the two middle long string with the hand level to the impact point.

Volleys

Impact configurations for volleys depends on how much time you have to prepare and how high the ball is when impacted. If possible take volleys at eye level with a racket that is at least 45 degrees above level. Most volleys should be impacted on the two middle strings with a neutral racket face.

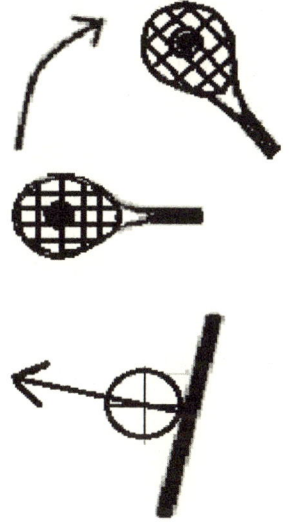

Catch and place every volley into the open court if impacted below shoulder level, unless you are deep in the court and have time to hit the volley like a ground stroke. Swing with more power and place every volley into the open court if impacted above shoulder level.

## Visualizing Impact Configurations

These impact configurations are commonly used by great players. Visualize one particular configuration as you are setting up for each shot. It is impossible to gain a powerful consistent world class game if you do not understand impact configurations. When I was young I was taught to visualize the ball going over the net and onto the court. That is not the best advice. Get into a good hitting stance with proper left – right alignment. Just before impact you need to visualize what you will actually be doing. You will be creating linear and rotational momentum with a chosen impact configuration. You need to roll the spot target as the strings are stretching. Visualize the exact spot on the string bed that you are going to crush through the balls' center of mass.

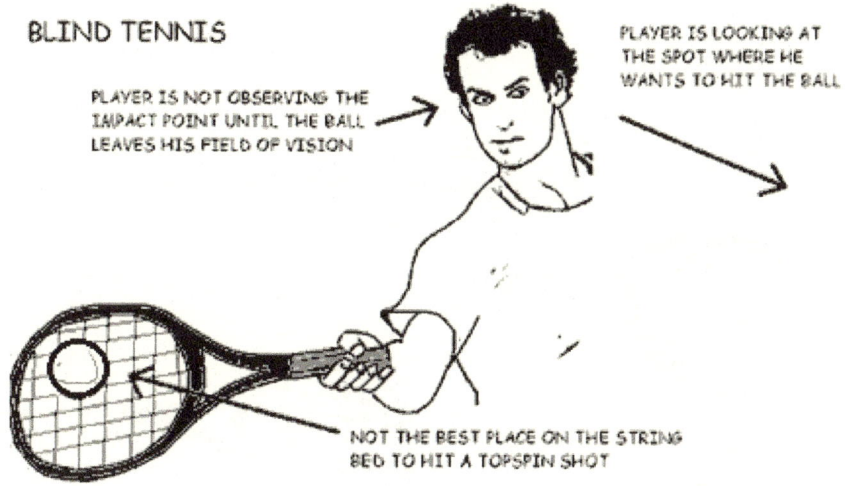

Your primary target is the ball.
Your secondary target is the spot you are hitting to.


If you believe that you must take every topspin shot on the two main strings then you will adjust away from the most efficient, most effective, and easiest way to produce spin if you are observing the impact. That is why many players end up pulling their head up. They rely on the feel of the shot for feedback. You must develop a feel for each shot. However, that is not the only mechanism used to judge how well you just hit a shot. You must use visual feedback and the feel of the shot together. The shot is not going to feel right unless it is impacted below the hand for topspin, above the hand for under spin, and towards the trailing edge for a spin serve.

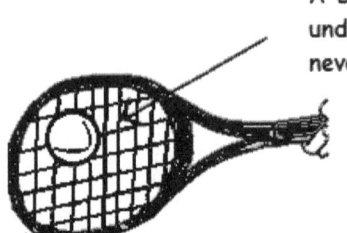

A ball hit in this location will put undue strain on the wrist and never have great topspin.

A ball hit in this location will have easy powerful topspin.

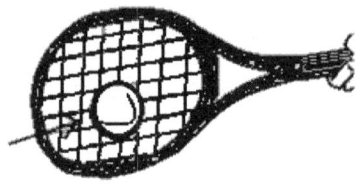

If you do not understand the string bed impact location and angle then you cannot visually adjust to that location and angle. This will force you to use blind feedback or never produce an efficient, easy, powerful shot. Blind feedback will eventually produce an above average shot. Only the use of visual feedback along with developing a feel for each shot will perfect your game.

You need all of your mental resources to actualize the best impact configuration for each shot. If you are ignoring these configurations then you are directing your mental resources towards a less relevant aspect of the game. Change the way that you look at the game. There are thousands of different locations, velocities, spins, and trajectories that you may have to deal with. Your best game is a slow to fast game. Move your racket slow until you are sure that you are going to catch the ball exactly as you plan to, then explode into to ball. This may mean that you are hitting some balls with a little less power. The control is worth a 5% power drop. Any teaching pro worth the price of a lesson will tell you that a shot hit at 100% power that lands somewhere near the service line is not half as good as a shot at 95% power that lands about 18 inches from the corner. Your long-term goal is to grip and rip with great placement.

Chapter 5

The Spot Target ~
A Simple Effective Targeting System

Aim for a small spot on the ball the size of a quarter or smaller. Keep your eyes on this target as the strings stretch into the ball. Smash this spot through the balls center of mass. This simple effective system is the very best way to aim the ball. Using the spot target does not take up any valuable time. It is also very easy to remember when under pressure. Aim for a small spot on the ball! Some players claim that you cannot use eyesight to see the ball when you hit it because it is moving too fast to focus on. They are half correct. You can see the ball and notice every detail about the impact. The ball is moving too fast to focus on.

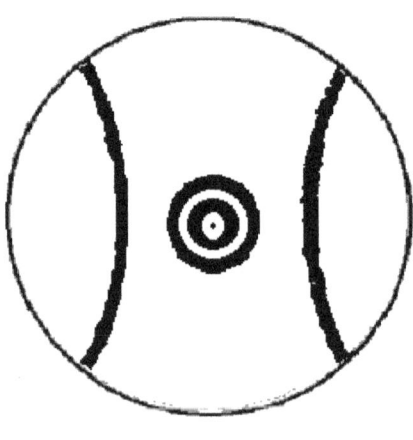

THE SPOT TARGET!

In order to best use your vision to your advantage you must watch every ball you hit as the strings stretch into the ball. In fact, the ball is too large of a target. You should aim for a small spot target on the ball that is no larger than a smart phone icon or a coin. Many players who adopt this method aim for a dot. The new trajectory should be created by smashing that spot target through the ball's center of mass every time. You need to visualize the first few inches or the first few feet of the new trajectory. Smash this small spot target through the ball's center of mass along the new intended trajectory every time. Even though the ball and racket are moving too fast to get a detailed focused view of the impact you still need to observe each impact as it is taking place and notice as many details as possible about the impact. This skill has always and will always account for over half of any player's success or failure on a tennis court. It is the most important skill in the game.

For a groundstroke hit without spin you should smash the spot target through the center of mass and impact the ball on the two middle long strings. The long strings and the cross strings should be perpendicular to the intended trajectory.

Average players follow the ball to the point where they believe that they can hit a good shot and then raise their eyes to look at the place on the other side of the net that they are trying to hit to. They are guessing where the ball will be at impact. This is the absolute worst bad habit in tennis. It is also the standard method that many people use.

Most players at every level are functionally blind at the moment of impact for each shot. People tend to get their feedback about the interaction between the strings and the ball by the feel of the racket. That is how blind people do things. They feel their way along.

The way a shot feels is a very important feedback mechanism. You need to add visual feedback to the mix. If you need proof of this then just look at any stop action picture of Andy Roddick as he is striking the ball. He is not looking at the impact. He is looking at the other side of the net. Compare this to any stop action picture of Roger Federer. He is looking at the impact every time. The internet if full of videos and pictures of world famous players. There are no pictures of Federer where he has pulled his head up to look at the other side of the court. Roddick had the most beautiful strokes in the world. He would look at the other side of the court when hitting the ball. Federer had the most visual discipline. His strokes look like a squash player. Their records speak for themselves.

Billie Jean King describes the basic tennis problem is that you have two targets, the ball and the spot that you want to hit the ball to. She correctly claims that pulling your eyes of the first target (the ball) is a frequent mistake that players make. A generation ago this was common knowledge. There are three reasons for this becoming a lost art.

The playability of modern rackets made it possible to play 4.0 or even 4.5 tennis without a proper visual strategy. However, without great placement made possible by a good visual strategy you will seldom get beyond club level tennis. Tennis is currently bottlenecked at the 4.0-4.5 level. Most players spend their entire life on the verge of great tennis and never get there.

Second is the modern teaching pro who typically stands in one place and feeds balls in familiar patterns. They probably undervalue visual skills because they could feed balls in their familiar patterns with their eyes closed.

The third reason is Vic Braden said that you are, "legally blind" to the impact. This is true. You could not read an eye chart if there was one printed on the ball. You are legally blind but, you are not functionally blind. You can see the ball well enough to notice every important detail about the impact. People who believe that Vic Braden's goal was to legitimize ignoring the impact, are misunderstanding him. Braden understood how peripheral vision works.

Any grown man or woman can knock the hell out of the ball. Power is not a problem for an adult player. Your goal is to knock the hell out of the ball and still control where the ball lands.

Following the small spot target while the strings plow into the ball is essential to hitting a good shot. The advantages of this basic visual skill goes way beyond the shot that you are currently hitting. You need to develop a basic idea of what each type of stroke should look like as the impact takes place.

The exact open or closed face of the racket, the exact spot on the string bed where impact takes place, exactly how the racket moves during impact, and where the center of mass of the ball moves as impact is taking place are all important. Once you start noticing these things then you will build up a frame of reference concerning the image of a good impact configuration for each type of shot and for each level of power. The impact configuration is the number one thing that needs to be visualized to produce a great shot. If you do not notice the exact impact configuration for every shot then you will have no frame of reference to use when you begin to hit each type of shot.

Many players will only begin to watch the strings impact the ball if they are behind or playing an important point. This is a mistake because every impact that you observe helps you understand exactly how to hit each ball. You will never hit the same shot twice. You must observe every interaction between the strings and the ball.

I have heard some coaches tell their player to look at the top of the ball. I disagree. You're going to hit a spot on the ball. Look at that spot.

The impact configuration is as important as all other details combined. The one group of players who watch the ball all of the way to the impact more than any other group are the Grand Slam Champions.

About 1% or less of all tennis players use their vision as their most important stroke production feedback mechanism. That 1% are always great players at any age, gender, or level. Visualize wearing the racket, "like a glove with no fingers". Target every ball as the string stretch.

Chapter 6

# Hold Your Focus on the Impact Point After the Ball has left the Strings.

Cybernetic: A goal seeking, feedback analyzing, self-adjusting system. A cybernetic approach to tennis visual and targeting skills is needed if you want to realize your potential.

Holding your focus on the point in space where the impact took place is the only way to gain visual feedback about each impact. You need this feedback to adjust your impact setup and aim to a small spot. In order to use visual feedback, you must understand how your eyesight works.

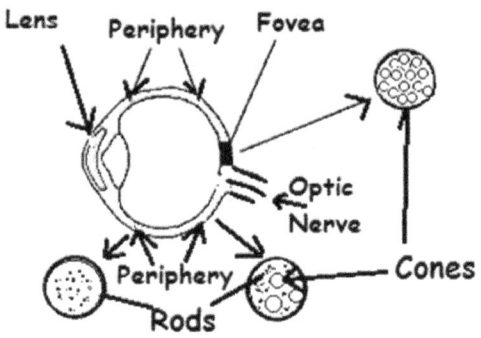

Vision is created with two mechanisms, focal and peripheral. The receptors that gather light for focused vision are called cones. Cones are designed to view stationary focused detail. The receptors for peripheral vision are called rods. Rods are designed to track unfocused movement.

Chapter 7

# The Most Important Tool That a Player Has

Light is focused by the lens on the Fovea. The Fovea contains only cones and creates focused detailed color vision of stationary or slow moving objects.

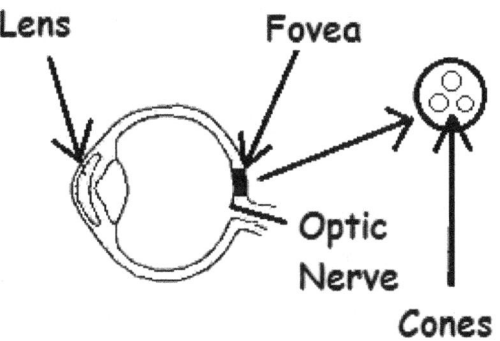

If you try to focus on the entire ball your eyes will never be able to focus as the ball is moving. It is better to focus on a small point in the middle of the ball. This is your, "spot target".

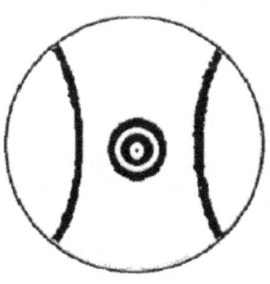

**THE SPOT TARGET!**

For the purpose of tennis your eye is a mechanism with lag time and limitations. Light enters through the lens and is not processed by the brain into a visual image instantly. It takes a few microseconds for an image to form from the series of electrical impulses that the eye sends to the brain along the optic nerve.

This lag time is very, very, very short. The impact takes place very, very, very quickly. A rapidly moving ball will leave your field of vision before your brain can process the information. The other limitations on your optic mechanism have to do with your ability to focus. Your peripheral vision will always be blurry. It is never in focus. This unfocused visual tool can track a very rapidly moving object. A rapidly moving object very close to you will never be in focus. It is not physically possible to get a detailed focused image of the impact. The most important instant in tennis can only be seen as a blurry image. That blurry image takes longer to process that it does to hit a tennis ball. Observe the impact any way. You can still tell exactly where the ball impacts the string bed. You can still tell if the long strings are exactly 90 degrees to the intended new trajectory.

You can still tell how to crush the spot target through the ball's center of mass. You can still tell the open, closed, or neutral face angle of the racket. You can still see the new flight line of the ball and where the balls center of mass moves as the impact takes place. You can notice every impact detail if you will simply stop ignoring the impact.

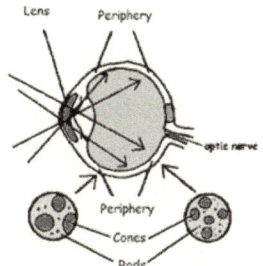

**Blurry Peripheral Vision**

The lens directs unfocused light to the periphery of the inside of the eye.

The periphery has larger cones that are far apart. The periphery also has Rods.

Impulses sent by the rods allow the brain to create blurry vision that tracks movement.

In order to use your peripheral vision to your best advantage you must focus on a fixed object and notice the movement out of the "corner of your eye."

There is no bio-mechanical reason to hold your focus on the impact point until the follow through is complete. There is a very sound cybernetic reason to hold your focus until your brain processes an image of the impact. The greatest players in the world all tend to use their peripheral vision as a stroke production visual feedback tool. This feedback tool is the secret to their magic. The concentration and visual discipline required to notice the impact details are the most important skills that a player needs. I have known players who would sell their soul for better skills. That's not ever going to work because no one is buying. The fastest way to great tennis is hard work, grinding practice sessions, respect for the response modes, patterned play, and most important is world class visual skills and concentration.

## Chapter 8

## Make the Magic:

Try this simple exercise. Look up from this book. Fix your gaze on the nearest door knob. If there is no nearby doorknob then pick some other small object at least 5 feet away. Extend your arm and move your hand across your line of sight. Move it past the doorknob and move it palm first. Do not take your eyes off of the doorknob. Notice the blurry ghost-like image of your hand as it passes in front of the doorknob. Do this several times keeping your gaze fixed on the door knob. Use the palm of your hand as a model of the racket, or use a racket. Quickly move your palm across the line of sight to the doorknob with a closed face and intersect the image of the doorknob low on the string bed. As you can see (not clearly) you can notice the exact orientation between your hand and the door knob.

The end-all, be-all, visual technique that will perfect your game is to follow the spot target on the ball all the way to the impact. Crush and roll the spot target. As the impact takes place focus on the impact point for just an instant after the ball has left your field of vision. This will allow you to holistically read the impact configuration. If you do not hit your intended shot then adjust one of the adjustable variables about the impact configuration or adjust your power level. The adjustable variables will be covered in the next chapter.

To use your peripheral field of vision to your best advantage you must focus on a fixed point and then notice the moving objects out of the corner of your eye.

This fixed point will be the impact point. Focus on the impact point until the ball has left your peripheral field of vision. This is not a trick or a gimmick. Your eyes are designed to focus on one point and notice the rest of your field of vision out of the corner of your eye. You will see a blurry vision of the ball and the racket.

The most important skill that you can develop is to gain information from this blurry image. Notice the exact interaction of the strings and the ball and compare this to the spot where the ball landed, the height that it cleared the net, the speed of your shot, and the amount of spin on the ball. Every time that you do this you will get better at adjusting your game.

Most people believe that keeping your head down and your eyes focused on the impact point until after the ball has left your field of vision is intended to ensure that you do not take your eyes off of the ball before you hit it. This is true, but it is not the entire story. When you keep your focus on the impact point after the ball has left the racket a really magical hidden advantage emerges. The exact orientation of the string bed and the ball's incoming trajectory become obvious to your peripheral vision. The exact location of the ball on the string bed and the exact flight line of the ball after it is struck also become obvious.

Even though it is a blurry ghost like image, you can exactly notice all of the most important things that you need to on each shot. You will use this feedback on your next shot to adjust one of the adjustable impact configuration details, if that is necessary. This will perfect your placement, power level, and spin imparted to the ball. The system for tracking the ball and the racket is the most important thing that you must learn. Make that mental switch from concentrating on the path of the racket to concentrating on the new path of the ball as you are hitting it.

You must choose one thing as your center of mental focus. Your ability to concentrate works much like your ability to focus with our eyes. Your eyes can focus on one small object at a time. You can notice other things out of the corner of your eye. You can concentrate on one thing at a time. Everything else must be in the back of your mind.

Before you were born, when you were in your mother's womb, your eyes and your brain were one organ, your eyes were part of your brain. It is no surprise that in terms of focus and concentration, your eyes and brain work much alike. The exact choreographed stroking technique is designed to create a particular impact configuration. The strings meet the fuzzball at impact. Choose to focus on the impact. Build your stroke and follow through around the impact.

This instant feedback is the best control tool that a player has. Crushing the spot target through the center of mass is a simple effective targeting system that will shrink the area that you can hit the ball to. Noticing the impact variables will perfect your control of the entire game. Better control means that it is easier to control placement, spin, and of course power. If you understand what is happening during the few microseconds when the strings are on the ball then very soon you will be able to get to the point where you can consistently use a slow too fast stroke to throw the racket through the ball as fast, as relaxed and, as powerful as possible.

Everything that you do to improve as a tennis player must take this vision technique into account. Build you game around eye discipline.   Use a check point sequence every shot. 1. Visualize a specific impact configuration as you are tracking the ball to the string bed.  2. Smash the small spot target on the ball thru the balls' center of mass along the new intended trajectory. Roll the spot target as the strings are stretching. Watch this happen.  3. Recall the exact interaction between the strings and the ball. 4. After you recall how the strings and ball interacted pull your head up and examine the results. This should take a microsecond and the ball should be somewhere near the net when you pick your head up, Notice the trajectory, the spin and most important; notice where the ball lands.  5. Adjust each stroke to perfection.

Make this the center of your game if you want to be a great player.  Make what the stroke looks like the center of your game if you want to be above average.  Use good form forehands to practice your targeting system and visual feedback technique. Use good form backhands to practice your targeting system and visual feedback technique. Use good form serves to practice your targeting system and visual feedback technique. Use good form drop shots to practice your targeting system and visual feedback technique.  Etc., etc., etc....

There are several hidden advantages to a visual feedback approach to tennis. Your strokes will tend to improve because you will miss hit fewer balls. You will be able to control more power and to place a powerful shot more accurately.

Soon you will be able to tell exactly where your shot will land as soon as you are hitting the ball. You must respect the response modes, and the Champions Pattern. These will be explained in later chapters. The response modes and the Pattern will help you recognize an attack opportunity. With proper targeting and feedback skills you should be able to really gouge on each and every shot from the attack zones and you should be able to place the full power shots to a very small part of the court with no errors!

Develop this skill. It doesn't take that long to master. Once you see the value of a simple effective targeting system and instant feedback about the exact interaction between the strings and the ball it will be easier.

It can be stressful to give up your old ways. Most people believe that their way of doing things is the smartest way to do things. Many people use the poor strategy of pulling their head up and looking at the point where they want the ball to go because it works better than anything else that they have ever tried. The problem with the Blind Tennis aiming system is that it leads to too many errors. You cannot control the ball when it is on the other side of the court. Visualize and concentrate on what you can control.

It is often difficult to change your game if you cannot see the value of the new method. Improving your visual skills will have an immediate impact on your game. This will make it easier to incorporate into your collection of tennis skills. You can only control what you are actually doing. A blurry view of what you can control is better than a focused view of the other side of the net.

Soon after you begin comparing the results of each shot with the exact interaction between the strings and the ball, you will be a great player. You must focus on a point in space that has nothing there. This point was the impact point. Hold your focus on the impact point and pay attention to your blurry vision. Notice the blur that is the ball and the blur that is the racket. This is tricky at first but it is a far superior method of gaining feedback about your shots.

Many people have been taught to keep their face pointed at the impact and this did not help. Following the ball all of the way to the impact is no better than pulling your head up if you do not notice every detail about the impact and use this feedback to perfect your game. This takes about a tenth of a second. It's really pretty simple and not all that difficult.

The absolute best that you can do is to RECALL the exact interaction between the strings and the ball on every shot. Discipline yourself to hold your focus until you process all that your blurry vision can tell you. Placement will be perfected. Errors will be quite rare. You will soon develop the reputation of being a tennis genius. This will happen very quickly. If anyone doubts that Roger Federer uses this or a similar system then I don't know what sport you have been following for the last 20 years. Stop looking at Roger's strokes. If you want to copy his success then visualize the racket as an extension of your hand. Look at his eyes.

Chapter 9

## Tennis Cybernetics

Learn the six adjustable variables and use them if you make any error. Holistically read each impact. Pay more attention to the adjustable variables if you are making errors. The adjustable details about each impact are:

Important for spin production:
1. The exact spot on the string bed where impact takes place.
2. The exact open, closed, or neutral impact angle relative to the incoming trajectory.

3. The direction that you are going to roll the spot target while applying linear force.

Important if you are miss-hitting the ball:
4. The exact spot on the ball that you are going to crush through the center of mass along the new flight line.
5. The 90-degree angle between the long strings and the trajectory.

Important all around and for power:
6. The spot right in front of you where you are going to, "throw the tip of the racket" towards.


You should recall each impact in a holistic fashion. Very soon after you begin reading each impact you will be able to tell where the ball is going to land as soon as you hit it and before you take your eyes off of the impact point. If you do not hit the intended shot with the intended spin then you should concentrate on specific items.

Practice the most important skills in tennis.

The six adjustable variables all need to be understood on an automatic basis. They must become habit. Stick with these exercises or develop your own to help you practice your feedback and adjustment skills. The best way to develop these skills is to drop hit balls at full power and read each impact. Adjust one variable at a time. Notice the effect of this adjustment. Eventually you will develop a holistic visualization for each type of shot. Keep in mind that you must adjust against every opponent, every day, every time you step on the court. Very quickly you will have world class placement. Hold your focus on the impact to holistically read each impact. Paying more attention to the adjustable variables will perfect your placement. The adjustable impact details are:

1. The exact spot on the string bed where impact takes place. Notice this every time. You should be visualizing the string bed impact spot for each type of shot. Very quickly you will find your favorite impact locations for spin serves, topspin, under-spin and shots without spin. The shot will feel right when you have found your favorite impact location. There is no need to practice this. Just visualize and notice the impact location on every shot that you hit. Adjust to your best location for each shot. There is typically not a need to use string bed impact location as an adjustable item when the ball is up. Find your favorite locations and stick with them. Dead center of the sweet area for volleys and spin-less shots. Favor the trailing edge of the sweet area for any spin shot. Explode into the shot when you are sure that you are going to use the exact spot on the string bed that you want to use to crush the ball.

2.     The exact open, closed, or neutral impact angle relative to the incoming trajectory.  This is the number one way to adjust the depth of your shots.  This adjustment really needs to be practiced.  You can begin by drop hitting balls.  This skill will transfer to a rally or point situation very easily.

Drop hit a full power forehand, hold your focus and, read the exact open, closed, or neutral impact angle relative to the trajectory.  Notice where the ball lands.  If you want the ball to go deeper then drop hit another ball.  This time try to keep as many of the other variables the same and open up the impact angle just one or two degrees.  Close the racket face a little if the ball is too deep.

Do this for several shots.  If you keep comparing the feel of the shot, and the visual feedback of the impact angle to the spot where the ball lands then very quickly you should be able to direct the ball to a very small area of the opposite court.  Practice this for all ground strokes.  It takes a very small adjustment to move the spot where the ball land a few feet deeper.  If you get good at this then you should be able to place most stokes into the corner of the deepest 1/8th of the other side of the court.  You should not need more than a two-foot margin of error.

3. The direction that you are going to roll the spot target while applying linear force.

This comes naturally to most players with any experience at all. Make sure that you are rolling the spot target when the strings are stretched. Compare the feel and the outcome for every shot.

4. The exact spot on the ball that you are going to crush through the center of mass.

This is the humungous one. The spot target should be crushed through the center of mass along the new trajectory every time. Most players like to aim for a spot along the new trajectory as little four inches or as much as two feet from the spot target. This is the number one way to adjust the ball to the left or right. You can also slightly raise or lower the spot target to help control the depth.

Crushing the spot target through the center of mass and controlling the open, closed, or neutral impact angle are the two most important variables that deal with adjusting your placement. Make sure that the long strings are 90 degrees to the intended trajectory. This really needs to be practiced. You can begin by drop hitting balls and hitting full power shots. This skill will also transfer to a rally or point situation very easily.

Drop hit a full power forehand. Aim for a specific spot on the ball. Crush this spot through the ball's center of mass. Hold your focus and read the exact beginning of the new trajectory when the strings are on the ball. Notice where the ball lands. If you want the ball to go to the left or right then make sure that the long strings are at 90 degrees and move the spot target just a little bit when you drop hit the next ball. This time try to keep as many of the other variables the same. Do this for several shots. If you keep comparing the feel of the shot, the spot target, and the visual feedback to the spot where the ball lands then very quickly you should be able to direct the ball to a very small area of the opposite court. For any given alignment you can easily hit a full power shot about 11 degrees left of right. If you are not using an aiming system and are trying to adjust the location by adjusting your stroke you cannot be more accurate than about 11 degrees. You should be accurate to within less than a degree every shot.

The two most important things about each shot are line and net clearance. It is very difficult to plan and execute an exact parabolic trajectory. Better to visualize the line. It is very easy to hit an exact line if you use the spot target. Once you are hitting your line it is very easy to dial in the rest of the shot.

5. The 90-degree angle between the long strings and the trajectory.

This is the definition of a cleanly hit ball. After each miss hit you must concentrate on making sure that every impact is 90 degrees to the long strings. This is true for any string bed impact location.


6. The spot right in front of you where you are going to, "throw the tip of the racket" towards and the exact arc that the racket tip follows.

This is the other humongous one. In order to hit a relaxed powerful shot you need to throw the racket through the ball. The only difference between actually throwing the racket and stroking a tennis ball is that instead of letting go you hold onto the racket. Two things will perfect your technique and control of the shot. The arc that the tip makes as it strokes the ball and an imaginary point in space just in front of you where you are going to throw the tip of the racket towards. If you pick this point on every ground stroke and serve then you will have another great tool to adjust a full power shot. This spot should be two or three feet in front of you and somewhere between your chest and head in height. For a windshield wiper right handed forehand throw the tip in front of your left shoulder, about shoulder height. This variable is adjusted by moving the tip target slightly up or down.

If you target and adjust this spot with your racket tip every time you will almost immediately become very good at hitting a full power normal shot. Pick the tip target. Notice the arc. Adjust the tip target to control a full power shot. Normalize Grip and Rip.

Tennis is all about adjustments. Do you have a simple, effective, immediate adjustment tool for a full power shot? By paying attention to where you are throwing the racket tip as you are watching the impact you can dial in a full power shot. After just a few shots most players have an, "ah ha" moment because they realize that they are visualizing where they are, "throwing the power." This imaginary point where you, "throw the power" will allow you to gouge on more shots with confidence. Throw the racket tip to an imaginary point. Move the point to adjust your shot. The visual feedback for this variable is the outcome of the shot. This will accelerate your development.

You should recall each impact in a holistic fashion. If you do not hit the intended shot with the intended spin then you should concentrate on specific items. It takes most players 30 to 60 practice sessions to develop a new skill as a habit.

Isolating these skills and practicing them is good. However, you should keep in mind that this needs to dominate how you think about the entire game. This is the most important habit that defines a champion. This will help as soon as you start using the targeting and feedback system. It will become second nature sooner than most skills because it has an obvious positive effect.

It is worth a few sessions to perfect your game. Your goal is to be able to cleanly hit every shot in a rally or game situation to 1/24 of the opposite court. For instance, if the ball is in the deepest 1/8 of your opponent's court and out of the middle 1/3 of the court then you are good.

The final visual skill has to do with anticipation and response. You should read each impact setup that your opponent or practice partner uses as they are hitting the ball. If you do this your anticipation will optimize. If fact every time that you watch a match you should be reading the impact on each shot. It is a golden skill. You can predict the area that the ball will land and in before the impact is complete.

It is commonly believed that you can predict with 95% accuracy where your opponents shot will land within a few feet after the impact. By holding your focus on the impact point and using your peripheral visual skills to notice all of the impact variables, you can tell almost exactly where the ball will land while it is still on their strings. This is optimum anticipation.

Chapter 10

## The Tennis Concentration Trance.

Develop a well thought out strategy for redirecting your attention when you become distracted.


Let's say that you are playing singles and you are serving. You should start to focus on the spot target when the ball is on your opponent's strings. You serve and volley, the return slowly floats to you at eye level. You plan to crush this volley into the wide-open court. Instead you take the shot for granite, lose your visual disciple, and shank the ball into the second row of the box seats. To make matters worse, your missed shot hits that super model that you were trying to impress in the face and spills her beer on the Queen of England. It was also a game point and now you are down 6-5, in the 5th set, to the Australian Davis Cup team captain. The guy from the racket company who was talking about sponsoring your next year on the tour gets "that look" on his face. This is not the biggest mistake that you can make. The biggest mistake that you can make is to let any of this affect your next shot. Smile at the super model. Bow to the Queen. Move to return the serve. Follow the spot target as soon as the toss is up and until you put away the next point. Make sure that you mention your great racket when the interviewer asks you how you handled such a challenging situation.

Your brain works like your eyes. Your eyes can focus on one small thing and you can notice several things, "out of the corner of your eye". Your brain works the same way. You can concentrate on one main thing and several things can be, "in the back of your mind".

Some people really believe that they can concentrate on two things at once. They are wrong. Try catching two Frisbees at once. Try drawing two pictures at once, one with your left hand and one with your right hand. It takes most of your mental resources to focus on one thing.

You must concentrate on the small spot target for the entire point except for the few microseconds that it takes to notice the impact configuration after you hit the ball. Everything else needs to be in the back of your mind. With a rapidly moving ball and a talented opponent trying to dismantle your game, you do not have time to think about anything else. The small spot target never needs to be in the back of your mind. You can focus on several things in sequence and even at a very rapid rate. Concentration is the ability to give your attention to one thing. Trying to concentrate on two things at once is the definition of being overwhelmed. Many 4.0 - 4.5 players are trying to concentrate on 5 or 6 things at once. It will never work. This is a very real reason why a fixation on what a shot looks like keeps many players from reaching their potential. It is more important to focus on your target than your weapon. You have to choose. If you do not choose to focus on the spot target then you have chosen wrong.

The best tennis mental condition is nicknamed the "Tennis Trance". The concept of a tennis concentration trance is inspired from transcendental meditation. The way that transcendental meditation works is that the person meditating will concentrate on one thing. Usually, but not always that one thing is their breathing. Anyone's concentration will eventually stray from that one thing. Often in just a few seconds another thought creeps into your mind. The skill that meditators will learn is to redirect their focus back to the thing that they are meditating on. When they are able to focus on just one thing for three or four minutes then they are getting very good at meditation. The ability to refocus your attention is the critical transcendental skill. It is also a critical tennis and a critical life skill. Redirect your mental state back to the Spot Target after each shot and whenever you are distracted. Again, it is the ability to redirect their concentration after a distraction that is very valuable to a tennis player.

The Tennis Trance is not a transcendental state. The ideal mental framework for tennis requires you to focus on the ball and use the back of your mind to analyze the situation. Tennis is a dynamic situation. You must think on your feet as you are focusing on the ball. You must realize that you will be distracted. When you become distracted, you must learn to refocus on the small spot target.

After each error that you make you must try to recall how the ball looked when it was on your strings. If you cannot recall what the ball looked like on the strings the last time that you hit it then you were not watching the ball as the strings created a new trajectory. On the next point make sure that you are focused on the spot target every time your opponent is starting to hit the ball. Follow that spot target until the ball leaves your strings. Recall an image of every impact.

Another very important time to redirect your focus to the spot target is when you have just hit an ace or a great shot. Do not be obsessed with trying to hit an even better shot next time. Many aces and great shots are followed by double faults and miss-hits. Refocus after each point and keep refocusing on the spot target throughout your tennis career.

When your main focus is the ball and all other thoughts are in the back of your mind then you have formed the Tennis Trance. When you are watching every shot as your strings plow into the ball, then you have formed the Tennis Trance. When you can recall the image of every impact, then you have formed the tennis trance. Focusing on the ball while the back of your mind selects the shot, the impact configuration, the spot to hit to, and the power level to make sure that your intended shot is good is the only competitive skill that actually helps you win the next point. Rebuild your strokes in practice. Review your technique between points or games. Concentrate on the spot target when the ball is up.

Refocusing your attention on the ball does not always come easy. It is the only competitive mental skill that actually helps during a match. If you have not played in several days or weeks then you will be more distracted. It might take two or three sets to get to the point where you have refocused enough to produce the tennis trance. Remind yourself to refocus on the spot target over and over again until it becomes the center of your competitive mind set. Do this every single time you play. Do this every single time you practice.

You have one tennis brain cell. You must choose what to use it for. Do not practice your forehand. Instead, use good form forehands to practice your visual discipline. Do not practice your backhand. Instead, use good form backhands to practice your visual discipline. Do not practice your...etc....etc.....etc. Smash the spot target through the ball's center of mass every time.

Chapter 11

## The End All, Be All of Strategy.

You need to understand the value of "normal power."

Hitting every shot as hard as you can is a strategy called BFMI. It stands for Brute Force Mass Ignorance. In typical boneheaded fashion, BFMI is the instinctive approach to the game. The problem with BFMI is that it is more effective against lesser players and less effective against better players. That is why you should use the automated, "Champion's Pattern" against all opponents even if brute force will beat them. You will resort to the familiar when under pressure. Normal Power in the pattern must be your go to. Normal Power is the power level where you make no unforced errors and hit the ball to a certain area of the opposite court. Depending on the players stage of development Normal Power is typically 60% to 95% as hard as they can possibly hit. The concept of normal power is the beginning and the end of singles strategy. The perfect player would hit the perfect shot every time. The perfect shot would win the point every time. The perfect shot and the perfect player are both imaginary. One sure way to really screw anything up is to try to do it perfectly. If you have a great shot at your disposal then you must pick and choose when to use it. A shot that might go in is not a reliable shot. In the entire history of the game not one single shot beyond the line or into the net has ever won an honest point. Normal shots at normal power wins matches.

A weakness is not a shot that is hit at less than full power. A weakness is a shot that cannot be relied upon to get the ball over the net and to a certain spot at normal power under pressure. If you are hitting shots that go in 75% of the time then you will lose 58% of all rallies where you have to hit three shots.

The really smart, really mentally tough singles player will define an offensive shot as one that is still rising after the bounce, when it clears the baseline or the sideline. You are not going to overpower a 5.0 or world class singles player for an entire match. If an opponent hits hard to a great player's best shot then they usually challenge them with a normal power counter attack towards their opposite crosscourt box or into the open court that is still rising after the bounce when it crosses the baseline. This controllable attack will often result in a return that can be attacked even more effectively. This is what blows a players mind the first time they play a world class singles player. Many of the great player's shots are not overpowering. The world class player makes very few errors and puts the ball in the right place every time.

The classic error that a young player makes in their first professional match is to try to attack with a down the line forehand from the baseline. This works against many really, really good players. If you try this against a pro they will respond with a full power deep crosscourt backhand or even worse a full power crosscourt shot that lands shallow. Then they are chasing a world class shot to their backhand.

Power also depends on how close you are to the net. If you are on the baseline it is usually not the right time to hit full power unless you really own your opponent, you own a big shot or you are hitting to a weakness in an attempt to unbalance your opponent. You do not own an opponent if you are in a close match. You do not own a big shot unless you can rely on it to go to a specific area of the court all the time. A shot with or without spin hit at normal power from the baseline will land on the court if hit with the proper net clearance. If you are inside the baseline when you hit the ball then the percentages are in your favor if you hit with more power. You cannot afford to rally from the attack zone.

The correct shot is situational. Great players find normal power for each stroke. This may be different for each match depending on what your opponents is hitting. Gage your normal power levels each match. You also need to gage your opponent's normal power level. If your opponent is hitting harder, then it will be easier for you to counter punch with more power and still get the ball in. If your opponent is hitting hard, then count their errors. If there are too many errors then they are not going to beat you if you get your shots in. Normal power is the key becoming a great player. The singles player should start off with normal power and adjust from there.

You will come across players who "Grip and Rip" and make few mistakes. This means that their normal power level is very high. There is no shortcut to achieving this. If someone hits hard and consistent it is because they earned their game in practice. Consistent power is good. Inconsistent power is the definition of a loser. You need to practice until you bring your normal power level up. You must remove all "flop" from your game. All great singles players have at some point in their development started hitting balls that go in every time. A dinker is a player who gets every shot in. Dinkers never donate points to their opponents. All pros are dinkers. All great players are dinkers who have practiced until they can dink the ball with lethal force. It is possible to make "Grip and Rip" your normal power level. This will take lots of practice and lots of proper technique. You really need to use the spot target on the ball to do this. Ignoring the fact that you are missing too many shots is not a good practice strategy. If you blast away at the ball all the time and then try to practice until your shots start going in, then you are actually practicing shots that go out. Champions typically raise the singles trophy by using normal power to beat a player who is making too many errors. Doubles champions know that power is more important in doubles than in singles. However, they still know when to trade shots and when to go for it. Trading shots is the singles mindset that wins matches.

Chapter 12

# The Four Response Modes

When to defend, rally, attack, and finish.

The four response modes are Neutral Rally, Attack, Defend, and Finish. The typical club player is always in the attack or finish mode. This is why they make so many errors. Some respect must be shown to your opponent's shots. Understanding these Four Modes will keep you in the point and win many points for you.

### The Neutral Response

This is big medicine with all mentally tough players. An automated neutral exchange is a directionally sound shot hit at normal power. A neutral exchange keeps you in the point. It is not a risky shot. Humans usually feel the need to get out of any pressure situation. A tennis point can be a pressure situation. The player who cannot handle the pressure will often hand the advantage to their opponent by trying to hit a challenge shot too soon. The ability to neutralize or counterattack a premature challenge by your opponent is the one of real secrets to winning many singles matches. Just use Automated Shot Selection and trade shots with them until they cough up an attack opportunity. If you and your opponent are of nearly equal stroke making ability levels then you will be able to engage them in a neutral rally for an unlimited amount of time.

It takes more mental toughness to stubbornly trade shots than it does to blast away at the ball. If you blast away then you feel like you are doing something about the pressure. You are. The trouble is that you may be losing too many points to avoid the feeling that you are under pressure. A neutral rally, in the Champion's Pattern, means that you are extending a pressure situation on purpose. The good thing about this is that you are extending the pressure for your opponent as well. Making the neutral exchange the center of your singles game means that you will get used to staying in the point.

Soon, you will not feel the pressure of a long point. You will be the pressure. You will dominate an opponent of nearly equal stroke making ability who overplays with too many premature attacks. The neutral exchange of shots is the type of play that all singles players must feel comfortable with. If you are using a good visual strategy then you will dominate a match against any player who likes to play long steady points and is not refocusing on the spot target every shot. Neutral rallies are lost when a player is distracted from tracking the ball. The modern game places less value on a neutral rally and more value on attack shots. If you are able to consistently weather an attacking opponent with a neutral rally deep to their corners, then you will destroy them because you are way above their level. If they can launch challenging attack and finishing shots from your attempt at a neutral rally then you must adopt a more aggressive game. Typically one or two shots deep into one of their baseline corners will present you with an attack opportunity.

The Defensive Response

If you are forced to hit on the run, hit a weak shot, back up to hit, hit from the open stance, or you are faced with any combination of these challenging situations, then you have been forced into the defensive mode. You are also on defense if you are forced off to the side of the court or way beyond the baseline. If you have been forced out of your chosen automated pattern then you will lose the point if you do not return to a neutral rally or respond with an effective counter attack. The goal of defense is to return to a neutral rally. If you neutralize their attack then it puts pressure on your opponent because their attack failed.

The best defense is a lob that forces your opponent back towards the baseline. Your lobs should go over the reach of a person who is at the net in order to make them retreat. Lobs are also used to give you time to recover. About half of all defensive shots should be lobs. If your lob is not out of their reach then you can expect an overhead smash or an attempted put away volley. You can also slice to the open court or hit at your opponent's feet.

A defensive shot keeps you in the point. You may have to play more than one defensive shot in a row. The defensive phase ends when you lose the point, are presented with a chance to counter attack or you neutralize their attack. Do whatever it takes to stay in the point. You may be out of position and be forced to hit a shot that is not in good form. If that is what it takes then attempt to impact the ball at 90 degrees to the incoming trajectory and work on your form later. Stay in the point and try to return to a neutral rally.

Defensive shots are lost because players are distracted by an effective attack shot and they forget to track the ball. Many forced errors would not be errors if better visual discipline was used.

The Challenge ~ Attack

An attack shot is a shot that is intended to unbalance, rush, or move your opponent. The ideal attack would force your opponent to hit on the run, not allow them to set up in a good hitting stance, and would be directed towards their weakest shot. The ideal attack would be hit from a good hitting stance, would employ a full backswing, be hit with all the power that you control, and would still be rising after the bounce when it clears the baseline or the sideline. Shots that can easily be hit into the open court or give you some other obvious opportunity to force your opponent out of their comfort zone are also attack shots. Effective attacks can be hit to your opponent's strong side. But, if you are given the option, you should attack their weak side. Although many times your opponent will not return an attack shot, the real goal is to force them to hit under compromised circumstances. This is an attempt to increase your opponent's errors and weak shots.

The extreme case of attack opportunity is the sitter. The sitter is a weak shot that bounces or floats "just right". The sitter is a ball that is presented to you in exactly the best location so that you can hit a shot that challenges your opponent to hit a weak shot, hit a shot on the run, or rush a shot.

Attack opportunities include weak serves, some mishits, shots that land in the attack zone, an out of pattern shot by your opponent, and sitters. You will be presented with some sitters every match. Every sitter is an obvious attack or finish opportunity. Attack them. Effective attack shots are the number one thing that wins matches. The player who hits the most put-a-ways does not always win the match. Opponents who make a lot of put-a-ways usually also make a lot of errors. The player who hits the greatest number of effective attack shots wins the match every time!

Another opportunity to attack comes when your opponent's attack does not work. If they hit a forcing shot but you have time to set up, you don't need to hit on the run, or it comes to your strong side then you can forgo any defensive ideas and hit an immediate challenging counter attack shot. Topspin forehands and slice backhands are often used to attack. You need to be able to attack and counter attack with a backhand as well as a forehand. Advanced players get very good at intelligent controlled attacks. If both of your feet are well inside the baseline when you hit a shot then you are in the attack zone.

The Finishing Shot

Finishing shots end the point in an obvious manner. You can "put it where they ain't" with normal power. You can smash it away. You can drop shot. The opportunity to finish will often come after you have hit a good challenge. However, it may present itself at any time. Many sitters can be placed into the open court.

Finishing shots are hit off of your opponent's shots that pose no threat at all. They are usually easy obvious shots and should be taken advantage of every time. Remember to use Normal Power at all times. However, Normal Power for a sitter about eye level at the net is about 150 miles per hour! Beware, you still need to watch the ball onto your strings, visualize the net and pick a spot over the net and onto the court to hit into. Even if a shot appears easy you must still focus on the process of getting the ball over the net and onto the court until the point is officially over.

Instant Karma

You must assess your opponent's shots instantly and decide on your response. If you think about the four main options and size up your opponent in advance then, your choices will usually be obvious. The player who hits the greatest number of effective attack shots will win the match. However, hitting Attack or Finishing Shots when the situation calls for a Defensive Counter or a Neutral Rally, is the definition of overplaying. Underplaying is where you hit a Neutral Rally type shot when you should have attacked or finished.

You are not always going to make the correct decision on the run. After each point that you lose there are two things that you must do. Try to recall what the ball looked like on your strings during your last shot, as you were hitting it. If you cannot do this then you pulled your head up. The second thing to do after you lose a point is to figure out if you chose the correct response. If you are typical of many players then you will soon realize that your mistakes are caused by over playing the situation or poor eye discipline.

Chapter 13

The Average Approach to Tennis.

The average approach to tennis is all about what the stroke looks like. You do not win points with a shot that looks good on a slow-motion video unless that shot can be hit in the pattern. Make visual skills, impact configurations, weight shift and mental discipline as important as stroking technique when teaching and talking about the game.

Most tennis players learn the game by learning stroke mechanics and watching pros play on television and You Tube. This is not a bad thing. They know that they are supposed to watch the ball but if something goes wrong with their game they look to stroke mechanics to fix the problem. Most players are so obsessed with the exact technique that they are distracted from the visual and mental discipline required to play great tennis. Making the form of a shot the center of your game is a great way to become an above average player who can direct the ball with an 11 degrees margin of error. You cannot concentrate on two things at once. If you are thinking about how to hit the ball then you cannot use the same brain to concentrate on the spot target or the string bed impact location.

The top players in the world all hit the ball with different mechanics. Sometimes the same pro will look different on each shot. Many players have beautiful strokes and make errors on far too many shots. Many average teaching pros love the idea that fixing someone's stroke is the end all be all of tennis improvement.

Sometimes it gets really absurd. I have seen pros and tennis websites absolutely dissect and analyze a player's strokes to find out why they are making mistakes. All the while, they ignore the fact that their client is not even looking in the direction of the impact. Trying to create a more consistent shot by adjusting the style and form of the shot while ignoring the visual and mental skills needed to hit a good shot will work after days of practice, but, it will not work right now. You might as well try to play a video game on your smartphone by using a ten foot wooden stick. If it doesn't work just get another stick.

If you are playing singles, then the tennis ball can bounce in over 5,000 spots on your side of the court before it touches the same spot twice, if you are playing doubles then it can bounce over 6,000 times without touching the same spot twice. The ball can come from several angles, with top, under, side, or no spin. The rate of spin can also vary from 0 to about 4000 rpm. The ball can travel from under one mile per hour to over 100 miles per hour. There are basically an infinite number of shots varieties that you and your opponent can use. How can anyone believe that there is one best way to hit the ball? Only when you start to build your game around the instant of impact will you be able to handle any variety of shot that comes at you. Wear the racket. Target a spot on the ball.

Did you know that preferring to repeat an exact motion over and over again is a symptom of cognitive impairment? Use your cognitive skills on every one of your thousands of practice shots. Do not impair your mental resources to stay in a mindless comfort zone.

Here are the nine most important things about each impact. They are in order of their importance:

1. Crushing the spot target on the ball through the ball's center of mass. Roll the spot target up to 12 o'clock for topspin, to 6 o'clock for under-spin, to 3 O'clock for a slice serve and to 1:30 or 2 o'clock for a kick serve. Crush the spot target towards the center of mass as you are rolling it.

2. The exact location on the string bed where the impact takes place.

3. Maintaining a 90-degree angle between the long strings and the trajectory.

4. The exact open closed, or neutral face of the racket relative to the incoming trajectory.

5. The weight shift into the ball. Create momentum by shifting your center of mass in the direction of the spot above the net that you are trying to hit to. Catch the ball on the strings while you still have momentum.

6. The amount and duration of pressure between the ball and the string bed. This is another way to say power level.

7. The arc of drawn by the racket tip and the spot that you are throwing the tip too.

8. The spot on the other side of the court that you are trying to hit the ball to.

9. The stroking technique for each shot. Yes, it is more important where you hit the ball than how you hit the ball.

The standard 4.0 mindset is to be obsessed with the 9th most important thing and to try and recreate an exact motion on each shot. 4.0 players try to automate their stroke production. Henceforth, the cognitive impairment that leads to the 4.0-4.5 bottleneck.

## Chapter 14

## The Champion's Pattern

Learn the basic singles game plan.

  Doubles and singles are actually two separate sports. Singles is an individual sport and doubles is a team sport. Singles requires pronated topspin first serves, normal power and automated placement selection. The number one rule for singles play is be consistent. Doubles puts more emphasis on slice and kick serves, power and service breaks. Formations are important in doubles. The number one rule for doubles play is be aggressive. Americans know how to play doubles with the best players in the world. Singles needs a fresh look.

  World class singles players understand that there is a definite pattern of play that needs to be followed most of the time. Great players automate their shot placement process. The "Champion's Pattern" is a common pattern used by NCAA and pro players. If you learn this pattern you will recognize it when you see a great singles match. Typically, the player who is able to execute in this pattern or force their opponent out of this pattern wins every time. If you automate your singles shot location selection then you will not waste time deciding what to do when the ball is up. You will hit the correct shot from any location on the court and you will appear to be a tennis genius to someone who is not using an automated secondary target selection pattern.

The biggest advantage of the automated target selection approach to singles is that it saves mental resources. You only have one tennis brain cell! Use that one brain cell to track the spot target.

The Champion's Pattern is used when you have an opponent who looks nearly equal to you in stroke making ability. If you can counter-punch their forehand from the baseline on a consistent basis then use the Champion's Pattern.

Shot Placement Selection depends on where you are on the court and what type of shot your opponent hits. If you use The Champion's Pattern against a player of nearly equal stroke making ability, who is not using automated location selection, then you are playing chess and they are playing checkers. They will have no idea how you beat them so easily.

The Champion's Pattern divides the court into two main zones and six smaller rectangles. The placement that you select depends on where the ball bounces. There are also two volley zones based on how high the ball is when you hit it. When using the Champion's Pattern, you should not attempt to win points with a great shot from deep in the corners. The goal of each shot is not to win the point. That is 15% tennis. The Champion's Pattern goal for each shot is to hit the ball over the net and to a specific place on the opposite court. The pattern will create attack and finish opportunities, if you get your shots in. Attack opportunities exist at any location other than deep in the corners. Normal Power, in the pattern, is your best game.

Always stick with this pattern if you can do two things. You need to get your groundstrokes hit from the Neutral Rally Zone into the opposite Crosscourt Box every time. You also need to be able to return their typical serves into one of your opponent's Crosscourt Boxes. The safest return is to your opponent's opposite Crosscourt Box.

The number one thing that you must know about the Champion's pattern is that there is a huge difference between hitting from the baseline to the opposite crosscourt box and hitting to the opposite 50/50 box. If you get the ball to the opposite Crosscourt Box then you will dominate because you will create attack opportunities. If your ball lands in the opposite 50/50 box then you are in the defensive mode and will probably lose the point.

This pattern is used if the ball bounces:

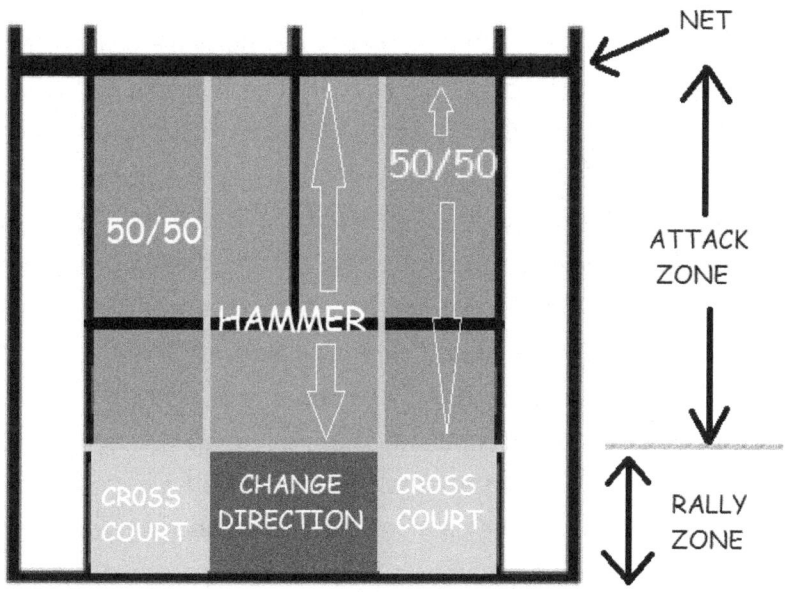

VOLLEYS:

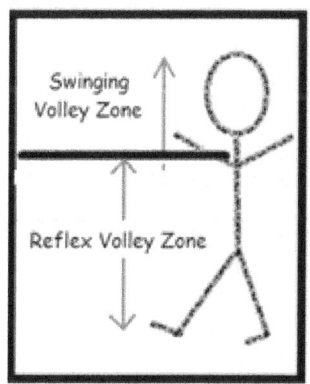

### The Neutral Rally Zone ~ The Champion's Pattern

If the ball bounces deeper than halfway between the service line and the base line, it is in The Neutral Rally Zone. Balls in The Neutral Rally Zone should be returned with Normal Power. Normal Power is the power level where you hit the ball to a specific location and make no unforced errors. Your ideal shot should bounce in the opposite Crosscourt Box, well inside the lines and still be rising when it crosses the baseline. This is not a power or attack zone. The Crosscourt Box can also be called the counterpunch box. The basic goal from the neutral rally zone is to counterpunch the ball deep to one of the opposite corners. Try to hit the ball into one of your opponent's crosscourt boxes. If that is not a comfortable shot then try to keep the ball deep. Remember, if you can consistently get the ball into one of your opponent's crosscourt boxes then you will dominate. Balls that are hit into your opponent's crosscourt boxes will often be returned into your attack zone. Keep the ball in your opponent's Neutral Rally Zone whenever possible. Every great player on the planet will counterpunch when the ball is deep, hit deep to the corners if that can be done with normal power, and wait for an attack opportunity. Every hacker on the planet believes that their strokes are so good that they can attack from anywhere on the court. Because they get away with this against weaker opponents they think it will work against a class act. It will not.

Crosscourt Box ~ The Champion's Pattern ~ Neutral Rally Zone

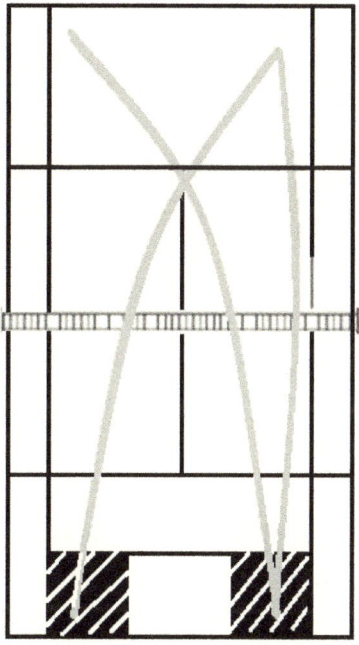

Balls that land in either Crosscourt Box should be rallied out to the opposite Crosscourt Box whenever possible. Be stubborn. Counterpunch any ball that your opponent hits down the line or crosscourt into your Crosscourt Box to the opposite Crosscourt Box every time. Keep them deep. You will win every match where you are successful in keeping the ball in the opposite crosscourt box. This will allow you to move less and cause your opponent to move more for each shot. A ball hit down the line from the Crosscourt Box is a low percentage premature attack at the open level, unless it is used to change sides.

You can use a high arching semi-lob down the line to change the side that you are rallying from. If you think that you match up better forehand to forehand then try to rally on that side. If you match up better on the backhand side then try to go backhand to backhand. If you can out rally your opponent off of both sides then you are going to win the match.

It is your goal on every service return to get the ball into one of the Crosscourt Boxes. Return into the opposite Crosscourt Box to start a neutral rally. Return into the Crosscourt Box right in front of you to attack. You will probably never be 100% successful in getting the ball into the targeted crosscourt box. Keep at it. Every shot that you hit into your opponent's Crosscourt Box increases your chances of winning the point because it increases your opponent's chances of hitting a weak return. Every shot that lands in their 50-50, Change Direction, or Hammer Box increases your chance of losing the point because it gives them an attack opportunity. This is why placement is just as important as power in singles.

Change Direction Box ~ The Champion's Pattern ~ Neutral Rally Zone

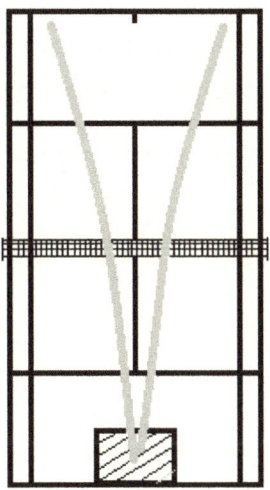

Balls that land towards the middle of the Neutral Rally Zone are in the Change Direction Box. Changing directions when the ball is hit towards the middle of the Neutral Rally Zone is a high percentage baseline attack shot that lesser players overlook. No great player ever hits to this location on purpose. You must take advantage of this high percentage attack opportunity. It is a good idea to hit the ball to the opposite crosscourt box when is lands down the middle. Many players will do this by running around their backhand and hitting to their opponent's backhand from this location. You do not have to change directions when the ball lands here. Changing the direction of the ball is your option if you chose to do so. You should choose to change directions every time that you have good alignment on a shot. Otherwise you are just letting your opponent off the hook.

Hit the ball into either of your opponent's Crosscourt Boxes from the Change Direction Box. It is recommended that you do not change direction on a very deep ball hit down the middle. Return all balls that are less than a foot from the baseline right back where they came from.

Always hit at normal power from anywhere in the Neutral Rally Zone.

The Attack Zone

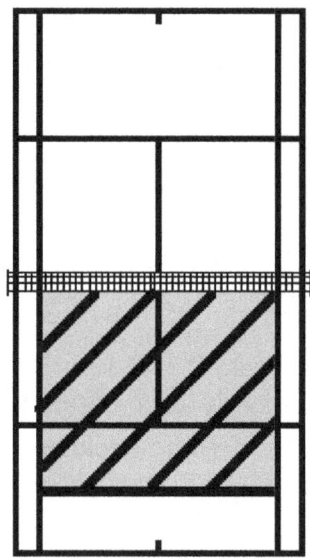

If the ball bounces anywhere between the Neutral Rally Zone and the net it is in the Attack Zone.

An effective attack is not a finishing shot. An effective attack causes your opponent to hit under compromised conditions. Effective attacks are:

1. Directed at your opponent's weakest shot. (Least risky)
2. Makes your opponent move. (A little riskier)
3. Rushes your opponent's shot. (Highest risk)

Typically, Normal Power is higher from the attack zones. Make intelligent attacks! Brute Force is not an intelligent attack if you do not hit a specific area of the opposite court. A normal power shot that is still rising when it clears the baseline or the sideline is an intelligent attack. It is even more intelligent if the shot is directed to their weak side, makes them move or makes them rush their shot. All great players do not underplay or overplay from the attack zone. Forcing your opponent to hit under compromised circumstances from the attack zone is the number one thing that wins matches. The attack zone is divided into the Hammer Box and the 50 ~ 50 Box

Hammer Box ~ The Attack Zone

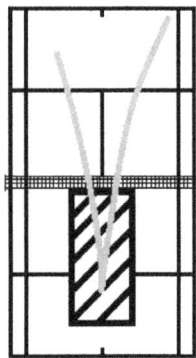

The Hammer Box is the strongest offensive location on the court.

The Hammer is defined as hitting your best shot to your opponent's weakest shot. Hit balls that bounce toward the center of the attack zone with a powerful groundstroke every chance that you get! When you hit a ball that has landed in the Hammer Box you should be attempting a decisive offensive attack. Make sure that it is an intelligent attack. Make them hit a weak shot, make them run, make them rush their shot, or combine these challenging situations to give you the advantage.

When you get a short ball that bounces near the center of the court then you have gained the advantage and must press that advantage. Your normal power level can be high from this location. It's Hammer Time! Pound their weakness or hit straight in front of you with your best shot unless you have a clear crosscourt winner. Now is the time to use intelligent brute force or hit an outright winner.

50/50 Box ~ The Attack Zone

The 50/50 boxes are very strong offensive locations.

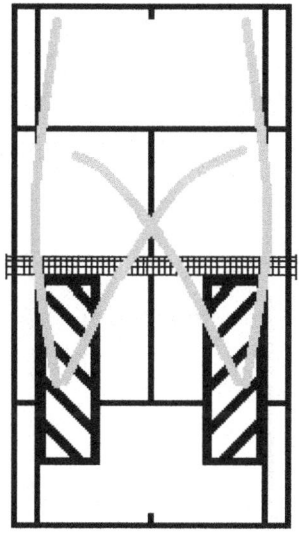

Deep crosscourt from the 50/50 zone is not a good option because will probably give your opponent an open court right in front of them. Half of the balls that bounce in the 50/50 box should be hit down the line and half should be hit short crosscourt. Your opponent cannot cover both. You will have the option of making your opponent run to every shot. Make them run or hit an outright winner. If the ball lands in your 50/50 box then you have gained the advantage. Normal Power is higher from the attack zones. Make intelligent brute force attacks or hit a winner. I often saw McEnroe use this location to his advantage. He would rally with his left handed back hand down the line over and over again until he got a shot that he could put away with a full power short crosscourt slice. It was a very beautiful part of his game.

Volley Zones ~ Champion's Pattern

Singles and Doubles:

The main thing that singles and doubles shot selection has in common is the volley selection pattern. Shot selection for volleys is not based on court location. Shot selection for volleys is based on the height of the ball when you hit it.

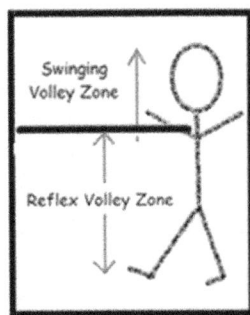

Swinging Volley

Above the shoulder is a swinging volley. If the ball is above your shoulder when you strike it then take a good swing at it. Make sure you clear the net and get the shot in.

Reflex Volley

Below the shoulder is a reflex volley. Punch the ball over the net and onto the court with normal power. Overplaying a low volley will lose you the point almost every time. There is no need to try and thread the needle with a 100 mile per hour shot. Your opponent will be rushed by any volley that goes in. Swing at the high ones and punch the low ones back.

Most players who have reputations as absolute gunslingers at the net have one secret. They guide a high percentage shot into the most open part of the court over and over again until they are presented with an easy put away volley or attack opportunity.

The Pattern Conclusion

Other Strategies

The most basic 2.0 - 4.5 strategy in tennis is containment. This mean that you simply keep returning each ball as deep as possible and wait for you opponent to cough up an out ball or a shot into the net. This is a defensive strategy and has some place in 5.0+ tennis. However, a 5.0+ player has a game and is not afraid to use it. Containment will not work at the 5.0 level for more than a few points. It is not enough to rally deep with a 5.0 player. You must rally deep IN THE CORNERS and respect the response modes.

The other common 2.0 - 4.5 tennis strategy is the backhand attack. This is also a less effective at the 5.0 level. Most 5.0 players have a great shot from both sides at the baseline and can hit any shot from either side along their chosen line. You can test each opponent to see where their weak side is. You cannot attack a weakness that is not there. If you can beat a player by attacking their weakness from the baseline then they are not at the 5.0 level or you are way above that level.

+1 is also a great simple strategy. What +1 means is that you realize that the first shots of a point are the most important. Plan on a killer serve followed by a powerful groundstroke deep into the corner. If you are returning then get your return in along a patterned line and attack the second shot. This is first strike tennis. This is great if it works. If both players are using +1 and you find yourself on the losing end of most points then the pattern is the best way to counter an effective +1 player. Neutralize their best shots. This will cause more errors and will give you more attack opportunities. Most shots in a +1 situation still need to be in the pattern. If the point progresses past the first three shots then get into the pattern. Try to force them out of the pattern.

There are a whole bunch of players who have reputations of being ninjas in doubles and total pushovers in singles. One of the basic problems with a 4.0 tennis player is that they play singles with a doubles mindset. Know the difference and play both sports well.

There may me an Idiot ~ Dummy guide to tennis. There is not a complete total Idiot ~ Dummy guide to 5.0 or world class singles. You have to be very smart to play great singles. Counter-punch strong crosscourt from deep in the corners. Every other location is an offensive attack opportunity that you cannot ignore. The closer you are to the net the stronger that attack should be. Change direction from deep down the middle with a strong counterpunch that makes your opponent move. Attack with more force if you are standing inside the baseline, catch and place low volleys, swing at high volleys.

Chapter 15

# When coaches blame their athletes

This chapter is entirely in response to a You Tube video that featured John McEnroe and Nick Bolliteri. The video inspired this book. In this video, both of these tennis legends blamed the recent lack of success that Americans have had as world class players on the athletes. My opinion of these two well-meaning legends dropped significantly when I saw this video. At one point in the video Bolliteri said something like ~"...the days of Jim Courier coming through the door are over..."

On the same day that I heard McEnroe and Bolliteri blame athletes for the lack of American success I went down to my local public courts for a thousand-shot workout. Right next to me were two young players who had been practicing for three hours. In my field of view as I was working out I saw about 200 young people who were involved in an all sports summer training camp. Each young athlete was giving it all they had during a High Intensity Interval Training session. I also witnessed one young person who was flipping a large tractor tire over jumping into the tire, then rebounding out of the tire with a 180-degree jump turn so that he could land facing the tire. Then he would do the same thing from the other direction. As I watched him jumping back and forth stopping only to flip this 200-lb. tire over and over again, it occurred to me that Bolliteri and McEnroe were full of crap.

The problem with American tennis is that we are lost in the 80's. We are doing the same thing that we did 40 years ago and do not know how to handle our lack of success. The players are blamed for a failure to modernize. Americans are very good at producing above average club players who look at the other side of the net when they hit the ball. American players tend to believe everything that they are told by TV announcers and advertisers. They are constantly getting the message that Americans cannot play great tennis.

Chapter 16

# Move Your Center of Mass into the Impact Point

This is an easy one. Early rotation into the shot is so 1980s. Just above your pelvis and in front of your spinal column is where your center of mass is located. If you are not in the defensive mode then what you need to do is begin every serve, ground stroke, and swinging volley by shifting your center of mass in the direction that you plan to hit the ball. This is true of all shots. However, is more essential when hitting groundstrokes with the eastern grips. Western grips still require a mass shift but they also require more rotation. Catch the ball on the strings while your center is still moving. This will create linear momentum and you can capture that momentum at impact. There will of course be rotation. The rotation will deliver the momentum at the end of the kinetic chain like the crack of a whip, not at the beginning of the shot. The weight shift should be in exactly the direction that you are trying to hit to.

Many people talk about a "racket lag". This is a horrible description of what needs to happen. The term "racket lag" tells you what you are not doing. What you need to do while your racket is 'lagging" is to shift your weight into the shot and MOVE THE RACKET in a spearing motion. A better term than racket lag would be, "spearing motion".

The racket does not lag as much as it moves in a linear fashion as if the butt plate were a spear point. If you begin each serve and groundstroke by attempting to spear the ball with the butt plate the normal course of the shot will cause the racket rotation to occur over a short period of time. Some pros call this, "pulling your shot." You pull the racket towards the impact. This will give the racket head more impulse to deliver to the interaction between the strings and the ball. This will begin the kinetic chain. Catch the ball just before the end of the weight shift as the kinetic chain is delivering its momentum.

Average players tend to over use the open stance and rotate into the ball with less of a linear mass shift. The linear weight shift along with a spearing/pulling early motion creates more of a rotation lag than a racket lag. One great way to learn this is to watch javelin throwers over and over. Use a spear throwing mechanism to begin your serve. The javelin toss is exactly like the early part of an effective service motion. The point where a javelin thrower releases is the exact point where the pronation snap should occur. After this makes sense to you, it will be easier to use a similar technique on your ground strokes.

This is one of the differences between doubles and singles. In doubles, you do not always have time to hit a complete stroke with a mass shift and the optimum use of the kinetic chain. Doubles players use the open stance more often than singles players. You cannot make a linear mass shift into the shot from the open stance. The open stance should only be used when you are in the defensive mode. The open stance should be used only when you cannot avoid it.

Chapter 17

# Linear and Rotational Momentum on the Ball

Momentum is created before impact. Momentum is captured and enhanced at impact. Rotational momentum is enhanced at impact by rolling the spot target as you are crushing it towards the center of the ball's mass.

Rotational momentum and directional momentum are two separate things. You must create both to hit a great shot. The outgoing flight path of the ball will vary depending on spin and power level. For topspin, you should visualize crushing the ball on a trajectory LEVEL with the court. This will create the linear momentum. Roll the spot target straight up the back of the ball as the strings are stretching. This will create a parabolic trajectory that is as small as 4 or 5 degrees and as much as 45 degrees above level. The new trajectory is created when the strings snap back into the ball. It seems counter intuitive to visualize a level trajectory. What you are really doing is visualizing the linear vector. The rotational momentum will alter this vector and create the parabolic trajectory. You will have additional control over the resultant vector by altering how closed the racket face is at impact. You have to create two separate types of momentum to hit with spin. Try it! It works! Crush the ball dead level to the court. Roll the spot target straight up as you do this.

This "windshield wiper" forehand will go in with as much force as you can supply. It is the most effective new shot ever devised. The secret is to visualize crushing the ball level with the court and rolling the spot target up as you do so. Adjust the open or closed racket face until all shots are going in.

Linear momentum is created by shifting your weight into the shot before impact. Linear momentum is captured and enhanced at impact. Rotational momentum is created at impact. The most effective rotational force is applied 90 degrees to the linear vector as the strings are stretching. You must visualize both vectors. This technique can be used to develop a full power normal groundstroke. In other words, if you have good alignment and you are not rushed you can hit a full power shot that will always go in.

When hitting with full power spin your arm's momentum and your entire body's momentum is towards the spot above the net where you want the ball to cross over the net. The directional momentum crushes the spot target thru the center of mass every time. Roll the ball on the strings as you are applying this directional momentum. You apply rotational and directional force at the same time. Great players can control a shot that is hit with as much or as little of both of these forces at once. Every shot is controlled by a balance of these two forces.

In classical mechanics, linear momentum is the product of the mass and velocity of an object. The linear momentum does not change that much when you hit with spin. You simply must shift your center of mass towards the spot that you are trying to hit to. This will create momentum. If you are hitting without spin then you must drop the spot target a few degrees below the ball's center of mass. You need to create a new trajectory that is above level in order to clear the net.

In physics, angular momentum (or rotational momentum) is the rotational analog of linear momentum. If you are going to apply a rotational force to the ball then you must do so as you are applying the linear momentum as well. Visualize what you are actually trying to do. You must visualize applying two forces at once in order to create an effective spin shot.

The linear momentum, does not change that much from a spin less to a spin shot. But that change is very important. You do not need to create lift with linear momentum when you create a topspin shot. A forehand topspin shot should be hit with a level linear vector. The roll and snapback will create lift. The spin will create a parabolic trajectory. A shot hit without spin and an under-spin shot impact the spot target at about the same place on the ball; just below level. The linear momentum for an under-spin shot and a spin less shot must create lift. Visualize a linear vector that clears the net. Roll the spot target as you are smashing the spot target through the center of mass.

Another reason why a fixation on the stroking technique is not the best way to approach tennis is because you are focusing on one thing. You must do two entirely separate things to hit a great shot. Visualize what you need to do.

Smash the spot target through the center of mass along your chosen line to create the linear momentum. Roll the spot target to create spin. Visualizing these two goals will help you hit a great shot. Impacting on the string bed above the hand for under-spin and below the hand for topspin have the effect of normalizing more power.

Many players have argued with me about this; until they try it. This is what a player learning or trying to improve their spin skills needs to know. It is also another reason why you need to concentrate on the impact. Your brains has the ability to effectively deal with one thing at a time. In order to deal with two things you need to rapidly sequence both events. In other words, your brain will switch back and forth between two things that you are trying to do. If you are trying to hit with spin then you need to deal with balancing two forces. You are basically trying to do something as difficult as catching two Frisbees at once. If you are concentrating on how the stroke looks on video then you are adding a third thing, making it the focus of your attention and placing the other more important things in the back of your mind.

It's the impact stupid! Everything else is decoration.

There are two entirely separate forces that need to be created to hit an effective spin shot. This is what players need to know if they are going to master spin.

The way that you organize how you think about the game is important. You need one mindset for practice and another for competition. Of course, you need to go from low to high with a proper stroke. Of course, how the shot looks is important. However, when the ball is up and the match is on the line you have to dismiss all distractions and focus on the spot target. Your simple effective targeting and feedback system are your top priority when a point is in progress.

Creating and controlling these two separate forces at once is the definition of great tennis.

The best analogy that I have is driving with a stick shift. The clutch and the accelerator must work together to get the car moving. Too much clutch, you stall out. Too much acceleration, you spin out. You have to balance the resistance with the clutch and the force with the accelerator. When hitting a spin shot it is often a matter of too much or little. Monster linear force and not enough spin and the ball goes long. Not enough linear force and the monster spin shot becomes a sitter. The ability to balance spin and linear force applied at different levels so that the shot goes into the opposite crosscourt box on a normal basis will make you famous.

Chapter 18

Roll the Spot Target

I know a Texas High School State Champion who credits a diagram very similar to this one for helping her win the state title.

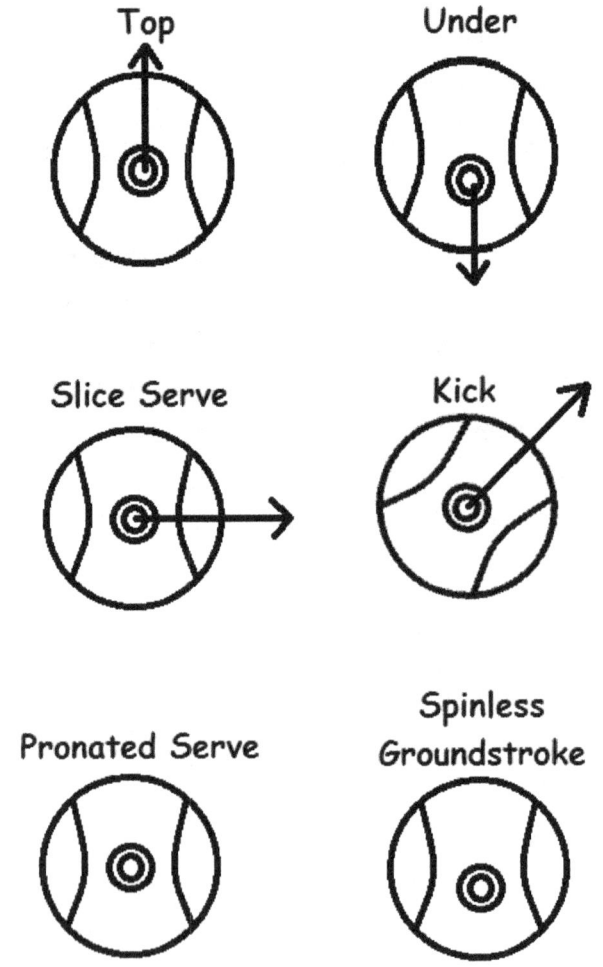

## Chapter 19

# How to Prepare for a Match

Develop a practice plan, develop a fitness training plan. Combine these to prepare for every match.

How to Practice

There are two basic types of practice, cooperative and competitive. Both are an essential part of a preparation strategy.

The Magic Number

The magic number for any athletic practice session in any sport is the number of successful attempts multiplied by the average pulse rate for the practice session. For instance, if you were practicing three point shots in basketball and you hit 45, missed 30, and had an average pulse rate of 120 then your magic three point shot number would be 45 x 120 = 5400. Another player who had 35 good shots, 40 misses and an average pulse rate of 180 would have a magic three point number of 6300. The second player would be progressing faster. Any sport requires you to perform with an accelerated heart rate. You must take this into account when you practice. If you hit 1000 good shots with an average pulse rate of 160 then your magic tennis number would be 160,000. This would be a better workout than a player who hit 1200 good shots with a pulse rate of 110. Their magic tennis number would be 1200 x 110 = 132000. The magic number multiplies the two most important things; successful attempts and pulse rate.

It is absolutely useless to have the most beautiful strokes in the world. You must have dependable strokes that can hit your target when your heart rate has been maxed out for 80 minutes. Tennis is a dogfight. Tennis is not a geisha dance. If you have a good practice partner who understands this then you can both attempt to engage in long rallies that allow both of you just enough time to set up with good alignment and hit an unrushed normal power shot.

Like all skills in life it is a balancing act. Make your partner move. Do not hit balls to your partner that they do not have time to properly set up for. If you both get the hang of this then you will both be great players. If you both want to be world class players then do this for at least three hours a day, three or four times a week. You need great cooperative tennis practice sessions, exercise, competition, and adequate rest.

When two champions go to practice they are more likely to cooperate. The smart player will pick a spot on the court to hit to that allows your practice partner just enough time to set up in a good hitting stance and hit a good shot at normal power. If their practice partner is doing the same thing then a situation develops where most of the practice time is taken up hitting balls instead of picking up balls. If this type of cooperative practice goes on for an hour then you probably will hit about 600 - 800 shots each. If you attempt to use 100% power then it will be impossible to get enough shots in or to avoid injury if you hit enough balls to really improve. Use long rallies and normal power.

Let the racket do the work. Really great players do not "muscle" the ball during long cooperative practice sessions. They build in slugfests as part of their practice routine. But during a cooperative session they take the ball in front of them and use the kinetic chain to make the easier powerful shot. It will take about three hours of cooperative practice on a regular basis to make you a world class player. You need to use a great stroke that you can hit all day long without tearing up your body. If you cannot figure out how to hit a good controllable spin shot with acceptable power that does not tear up your body then you are not smart enough to be a great tennis player.

The real trick to making cooperative practice work is the performance goals that you concentrate on. Hop step and track the ball as soon as it comes off of your practice partner's racket. Move quickly as soon as you can tell where the ball is going. Take big steps if you have a long way to go. Take small steps to adjust your position. Check your grip every shot. Gain a comfortable well aligned hitting stance when the ball bounces in front of you. Shift your center of mass towards the spot above the net that you want to hit to. Use a slow to fast motion to catch the ball with the chosen impact configuration while your weight is still moving forward. Focus on the impact point until you take note of the impact details. Use every shot to practice your visual skills. Holistically view each impact. Concentrate on the impact details if you do not hit the desired shot. Use good form on your backhands to practice all adjustable impact items. Use good form on your forehands to practice your visual skills and discipline. Use good form... etc....etc.... Lift the ball as the strings are stretching to put slow topspin on the ball. Use proper net clearance. Move the entire arm forward for the entire time that the ball is on the strings. Follow thru with your elbow at shoulder level. Recover to the line of most likely return. Assume the ready position when the ball bounces in front of your practice partner. Hop step and focus on the spot target when your practice partner is stroking the ball...

These performance goals will make you a great player. By backing off of power, using normal force and placing the ball so that your partner can return it every time you will be making these performance goals second nature. These performance goals need to be automatic. You will resort to the familiar when you are under pressure. When you compete you need to focus on the spot target.

I once saw Bjorn Borg and Jimmy Connors warm up for over a half hour. They were about to play an exhibition match in Seattle. They were still hitting the same ball at the end of the half hour. The rally never stopped. There was no love lost between these two great players. They were both using a slow to fast motion to get every shot in. It was obvious cooperation for their mutual benefit.

Cooperative Practice is the most powerful magic of all. If you focus on all of your performance goals for two or three cooperative practice sessions a week then it will soon become very easy to accelerate the strings through the ball a little faster to put powerful spin on the ball. It will help your offensive game and your counterpunching game because it will make your shots second nature.

During cooperative practice, you will be picking a spot over the net and on the court to hit the ball to. You will be focusing on your impact every shot. It will soon be easier to place the ball wherever you want it to go. One thousand cooperative practice sessions of one thousand good shots apiece will make you a great player.

Practice on a wall can also be effective but you must be careful. The wall will return all balls and this makes it tough to gage if your shot might have been in. You must do three things correctly when you practice on the wall or that practice will not transfer to better play on the court.

1.      You must use your imagination. If the ball is not coming down when it hits the wall then that shot may be out if hit on a court. Do not count balls that you think would be out.

2.      You must use proper string bed orientation. If you hit shots on the wall with the string bed at 90 degrees to the incoming flight line of the ball, then it will be easy to transfer to hitting on a court. Concentration on string bed orientation as outlined earlier will make practice on the wall very effective and will not throw your game off when you move to a court.

3.      You must use the wall to practice the visual skills. If you want to get real good at blasting away at balls hit to the wall and you don't care if it helps your actual game then just blast away. If you want your practice sessions on the wall to help your game then use the wall to practice your simple effective targeting and feedback system.

The Grind

The Thousand Shot Workout is typically called "The Grind". It is a sure way to become a great player. This type of workout was common when the Americans were dominating the tennis world. The Thousand Shot Workout is simple. You are going to hit a thousand shots in a cooperative setting. Do not count shots that go out or into the net. It is a million times better to use a count and only count good shots than to just go hit for three hours. Using a shot count creates a consistency standard. Americans ignore consistency. That is one reason why they are not much of a threat to world class players these days. This may take two or three hours the first time that you do this. After a few sessions, you should be able to finish a thousand shot workout in about an hour and twenty minutes. Here is an example of a good thousand shot grind:

Start out with 50 strait, 50 slice, and 50 kick serves. Mix then up to all 8 aim points. If time is limited then get a basket and serve side by side. If you have a couple of hours then have your practice partner return these serves. Do not play these points out if time is limited. Only count the serves as part of the shot count. Then switch. Have your partner complete 150 serves. This is the warm up and counts as 150. Then use normal force to rally crosscourt forehands for 150 shots each. Next use normal force to rally crosscourt backhands for 150 shots each. Then one player hits down the line forehand and the other does down the line backhands 150 each. Then switch to the other sideline for 150 more each.

Next go one up at the net hitting medium paced volleys and one back hitting ground strokes for 100 each. Then switch up and back or 100 more. Finish by hitting lobs and overheads 50 each. Let the lob bounce and hit an off paced overhead back to the lobber so that you keep the ball going.

There is not enough time in the day to complete this work out unless both partners are trying to cooperate. You can mix this workout up and change the number of shots that you hit of each type. Sometimes you can rally for 1000 shots and don't count any one shot. Never use this workout unless at least 700 of the shots are groundstrokes. The important thing is that you practice everything and you hit at least 1000 shots. If you and your partner are both hitting at normal power then you can hit a shot every 6 seconds. This means that you could hit 10 balls a minute. It would take about 100 min to hit a thousand shots. A good goal is to try and do this in 2 hours. If it takes longer than two hours then you are missing too many shots. Slow your racket down enough to get every shot to the best spot on the other side of the net. Talent is always trumped by dedication. Finish at least one Thousand Shot Workout between every practice match. Do not attempt to attack or finish. Do not try to force your practice partner into the defensive mode. Play a match between each 1000 shot workout. After each match find your max pulse rate. Then take a day off if possible.

You will need to build up to 1000 shots. Start out with a 300 shot count. After you have exercised, rested at least one day and, practiced or played in a competitive manner and then try another grind for about 500 or 600. Then exercise, rest, play and go for 1000. It takes a good practice partner to make this work. If you find a partner who is smart enough to grind with you in the correct manner then buy them lunch every once in a while and keep them on your Christmas card list. You are going to need each other to become great players. This drill is not called the grind for nothing. There is nothing recreational about it. The grind however is very effective in making you a great player! There is also nothing wrong with going for a 2000 shot workout as long as you get adequate rest.

The Thousand Shot Workout will groove the performance goals needed to turn you into a great player. If you work on the proper performance goals with cooperative practice then all you need to do in order to "Grip and Rip" is to add a little more acceleration thru the ball and a little more spin. Great tennis is played by those who have earned their game in practice. Any knuckle head can learn a forehand. A forehand does not make you a touring pro. If you have any real aspirations of playing at the highest levels of tennis then forget about it unless you are already a great player and you are willing to take eight months and hit about a million balls. That means five days a week hitting about 7000 balls a day. About 600 or 700 of those balls should be serves. The rest should be a good mix of all your shots.

Your arm and shoulder will fall apart if you try something like this without an efficient stroke. If you do not take a day totally off from all tennis and all physical activity every three or four days then you will never make it. You will also need to train and compete.

Becoming a touring pro is impossible. Those who make it have done the impossible. It is even more impossible if BFMI is your only method. I have met several boneheaded Americans who will not give up on BFMI and try a thousand brute force shot workout. None of them were able to finish the workout. Many of them are injured hackers.

The possibilities are endless. Use the magic number to evaluate any new cooperative drill or practice routine. Here are two examples of cooperative practice drills and exercises:

Thousand Ball Drop Hit – Grip and Rip – Cooperative One Person Drill

Get a basket of balls or a cart with as many balls as possible. Count the balls. Figure out how many times you need to fill the basket or cart to get to 1000. Run side to side and drop - hit shots from your crosscourt corner to the opposite crosscourt corner. Pick up one ball at a time from the basket. If done correctly this is better for your game than a 1000 shots hit on a wall. This drill will improve your placement and hand strength. Come to a complete stop with both feet planted.

Use proper form. Drop hit a powerful forehand topspin shot. Your goal on all shots except drop shots is to hit a shot in the Champion's Pattern that bounces in and is still rising when it crosses the baseline or the sideline. Turn and run towards the left side of the baseline. Pick up one ball as you move past the center mark. If you missed the shot then turn around after you pick up another ball and hit the same shot. If you make the shot then, run to the left side of the baseline, drop and hit a powerful topspin backhand. Come to a complete stop with both feet planted as you hit each shot. Turn and repeat until you reach 1000.

Take advantage of the fact that you have complete control of the situation and practice powerful ground stokes into the opposite crosscourt box. After you reach 1000 then hit at least 50 shots from every location in the pattern. Do 50 hammers, 50 from each 50-50 zone down the line and 50 from each 50-50 zone short crosscourt. Then drop hit 50 from both sides of the change direction box.


Volley Game vs. Courtney

This is a cooperative – competitive drill. Players should check their positions before each point to make sure that they are halfway between the service line and the net. The action is similar to playing catch. This can be a very advanced drill with four players. In order to win a point it is best to return each volley in a manner that will allow your practice partners to hit a standard volley without too many heroics involved.

Play "catch". If there is more than one person on the other side of the net then try to return each volley to the person who did not hit it to you. One person feeds the ball. In order to win a point every player must hit two good forehand and two good backhand volleys. Otherwise Courtney wins the point. All players on both sides of the net compete against Courtney. If a point is won then the drill becomes competitive and each player tries to put the ball away. The competitive part of the drill counts as well. It occurs after the point with Courtney is over. With two players then either player or Courtney can win. It's kind of like playing with three players. Let's say that Courtney wins two points, you have won three points and your opponent has won one point. The score will be 30-40-15. You can also play with one doubles team and one singles player or with two doubles teams. Play at least one set.

Competitive Practice

Competitive practice means that you are trying to win each point. This is the type of practice that resembles a match. The list of options for competitive practice is endless. You can play points, tiebreakers, king of the court, a set, or a match. Your coach can feed balls for a competitive drill. There is no wrong way to do this as long as you are simulating a match situation or you are actually playing a match.

The following pages contain several simulated sets and competitive drills that can be done by one person. Many players prefer these to practice matches because they have complete control over the situation. Many average players will only practice in a cooperative manner. Other average players will only practice in a competitive manner. Some average player will only practice their strokes. The best players will practice everything and spend time on rest and conditioning.

Here is an example of a one person competitive workout. You can use your imagination to make any ball drop drill or service practice a competition against a consistency standard just by inventing a scoring system. Practicing and keeping score against a consistency standard is how you practice handling pressure.

Practice Set vs. Wally

Basis rules:

The player will serve against the wall and rally. Two good forehands and two good backhands must be hit before a mistake is made or the point goes to Wally. Keep score like a regular set. Each shot must be judged based on whether or not it would be good on a real court. The dangerous thing about practice on a wall is that the wall will return all shots even if they would be long on a real court. The serve must be close to the imaginary net and going down. If the serve is five or six feet high and still rising when it hits the wall then is not realistic to believe that it would be good on a real court.

Calling a serve good or out is a judgment call based on trajectory and spin. The standard for ground strokes is dropping or rising. If a topspin groundstroke or a slice backhand is dropping when it hits the wall then it is reasonable to believe that it would be good on a real court. Like all practice on the wall string bed orientation must be concentrated on or it will be difficult to transition to a real court.

There is no penalty for hitting extra shots. It is best to go ahead and hit the shot that you are lined up for. The extra shots are considered neutral rally type shots and should be used to set up your required shots or to recover. There is also no requirement to hit the ball on the first bounce. It is more important to maintain good contact alignment and proper form than to take the ball on the first bounce. Do not hit the ball off the wall on the first bounce if you have to cramp your stroke to do so. Practice on the wall and tennis in general should have more of a badminton mentality than a racquetball mentality.

Advanced Standards:

Add a powerful explosive ground stroke to end the point. A good serve and two good ground strokes off of each side must be hit first. Then all extra balls must be judged as good until a very explosive forehand or backhand can be hit. It is best to maintain a neutral rally type of shot until a ball that is just right allows the player to explode into the shot. Spin must be used to control the final explosive shot. The all shots must be past the top of its arc when it hits the wall in order to be counted good.

If all shots, including the last powerful shot is good then you have won the point. You can rally out the ball for practice or catch the next shot and start another point. You will beat many good opponents if you beat Wally with these standards. Stay with these standards until you can beat Wally 6-0 every time.

Competitive Standards

Add other shots until the set is winnable but also a real challenge. An example of a competitive standard is two good topspin forehands, three good topspin backhands, one good slice backhand and then an explosive shot to end the point. The standard that each of these shots must be past the top of its arc when it hits the wall make this a very challenging drill. You are going to beat the daylights out of good players if you beat Wally with these standards.

The Ultimate Game against Wally

The Ultimate Game against Wally requires a good serve, two topspin windshield wiper forehands, two eastern forehands, three topspin backhands, one slice backhand, an explosive shot, a slice approach shot, a drop shot and two volleys off of each side. You must wait to hit your slice approach shot until you complete all other ground strokes. You should be at least halfway up to the wall when you hit your drop shot. For this drill you should hit the drop shot should go about as high as the top of the wall and be coming down when it hits the wall. Use the drop shot to come closer to the wall right after your slice approach. Extra shots at the net will sometimes have to be half volleys.

If you complete all four required volleys then you have won the point. You can catch the ball or hit the ball down on the court just in front of the wall and produce a lob like shot off of the wall. You can chase this shot down and start the sequence over again. If you can beat Wally with these standards then you should be able to play against anyone. You will beat many ranked players and you will make it interesting against the toughest opponents that you can find. If you are ever able to hit the lob type shot, chase it down, and restart the point over again, and again long enough to win a set without stopping then please contact me if you are ever in San Antonio. I will need you to be my doubles partner. Bjorn Borg is known to have played imaginary games against the wall as a major part of his early development.

Slugfest

Great players also need to have at least one slugfest before each match. This is considered competitive practice. What you do is to find a great partner and go ahead and hit every shot that you are lined up for as hard as you possibly can and still get the ball in. Do not hit to the open court. It is sort of like a grind except you use the most power that you can control. Hit into your partners strike zone with as much power as you can control. Continue until you are exhausted.

The Hoodie Drill

The Hoodie Drill makes service practice as aerobic as possible. The hoodie makes it a lot easier to get your pulse rate up. Fill the belly pocket of the hoodie with as many balls a possible. Put as many balls a possible in your pants pocket on your tossing side and hold as many balls as you can control. You are going to serve one serve after another without pause. Use the forehand volley position with the racket straight up. Do not use your windup. Just use the weight shift, the power stroke, and the follow through. By serving from the forehand volley position you can serve a shot about every three seconds. Do not stop to think. Just adjust the spot target until all serves are going in. This is very aerobic way to practice serves. If you practice in this manner it will soon become apparent that you are going to miss every serve where you have poor eye discipline and make every serve where you observe the strings impacting the spot target. This drill does not give a player time to over think. They have just enough time to adjust the impact. You should be getting one serve after another in. Try it. Start with 15 or 20 serves your first day. Add another load of balls into your hoodie each time until you are doing 150 - 200 serves per drill. If you have a pretty good serve that leads with the butt plate of the racket and resembles a javelin toss then this drill will BLOW UP YOUR SERVE!! It will create a very accurate, very fast, and very powerful pronated serve in very little time. After you finish this drill hit 15 or 20 serves with a full windup motion.

Practice and play against a standard for consistency is just as important as strength, stamina and stroke production. About ¼ of your time devoted to tennis development should be competitive practice. About ¼ of your time devoted to tennis development should be cooperative practice. About ¼ of your time devoted to tennis development should be devoted to conditioning and physical training. About ¼ of our time devoted to tennis development should be rest.

The set against Wally counts as competitive practice. This drill simulates the pressure of a real match. All simulated set drills are more about concentration, correct level of power and mental toughness than they are about stroke mechanics. So is a real match. Stroke mechanics and proper form are important but they are not the end all be all of tennis. The main thing that must be concentrated on when playing a point is the ball. Pick the spot on the ball that you wish to hit. Visualize the intended flight line of the ball for the instant that it is on the strings and then make this happen on every shot. This works when you play Wally and it works against real players. These types of drills and practice sets are limited only by your imagination. Make the drill a challenge and still keep it obtainable. The world is full of American players with great looking strokes who lose to smarter players. If you want to look good when you are losing then just practice what your shots look like. Don't be an All-American tennis bonehead!

Training:

The basic goal of every tennis player is to be, light, strong, quick, tough, and inexhaustible. Great players have found the right balance between exercise, practice and rest. You must train with as much intensity as possible and moderate that intensity to make sure that you do not over train. Power is the ability to apply force quickly. Power is the goal of any tennis training program. A champion must be able to apply power, and then reflex and apply power again very quickly. High or Medium Intensity Interval Training should be the center of your training strategy.

How not to Train:

Do not train to become big and strong. Train to become light and strong. Do not play and train 7 days a week. You have to manage your stress/rest cycle. Go light on the training on the day before a match. Do not train to be a bodybuilder and then try to make it work on the tennis court. If you want to train to be a bodybuilder then give up tennis and take up bodybuilding.

The worst thing that you can do is to go to the gym and do three sets of weights where you max out each set, work all muscle groups and make this a three times a week thing. Muscle recovery is not the problem here. Tennis and weight lifting both stress out your tendons, ligaments, and cartilages. If you train hard in the weight room and then try to play and practice you will develop overuse injuries. That is a rock solid guarantee.

When you are sore is usually not your muscles that are sore. It is your tendons and ligaments. The strength of these connective tissues is actually more important to a tennis player than max bench press strength. That is why the number one rule for all tennis players is to include a rest strategy in their training routine. Adequate stress plus adequate rest will lead to improved physical health and strength. Stress plus stress plus stress without rest will lead to injury. Your typical great player is not limited by their lack of strength. Greatness is limited by overuse injuries. If you do not need a day of total rest once or twice a week then you are not training hard enough. You must balance training, practice, competition, and rest. You cannot over train. Figure out what works for you. Your typical injured hacker believes that they are that special person who can ignore proper rest. They cannot. Your body grows stronger in response to stress only if it has adequate down time.

Classic Tennis Exercises

Jumping exercises are the classic way to train. But you must be careful. Think like a pilot. The most important skill is landing. If you fly a plane to Colorado Springs instead of Denver then that is embarrassing. If you screw up a landing it's called a crash. Jumping is similar. Most any jump is good for you. You must land as lightly as possible. Do not land straight legged. Do not slam your feet down when you land. DO NOT LAND OF A HARD SURFACE. If you make jumping part of your routine then find a good mat or nice soft patch of grass to land on.

You also need to be very careful with this type of training if you are injured, have arthritis, or you are getting on in years.

You can get into great shape without jumping. However, if you can safely work this into your routine it will pay big dividends. Under do it at first and work up to a more challenging routine. Any jump can become a tennis jumping exercises if your center of mass is dropping when you start the jump. Jumping as your center of mass is dropping creates explosiveness. Try all of these jumps. Use precautions and build up gradually.

Squat Jumps:

Place your feet shoulder width apart. Bend primarily at your knees and a little at your hips. Keep your back straight. Squat low enough so that your knees are at a ninety degree angle. As your weight is still dropping jump straight up and reach as high as you can with your arms. Bend your knees a little as you land and go right into the next squat. Try to land as gently as possible. Make sure that you jump over and over as your weight is dropping. Do not wait in the squat position. The reflex motion is what makes the magic happen.

Lateral Jumps:

Get a one square foot piece of cardboard and fold it in half like a little tent. Stand next to it sideways and jump sideways over the cardboard. Takeoff and land on both feet. Rebound from the landing right into the next jump. Go back and forth across the cardboard tent ten or twenty times. This type of jump is a great way to fake a poach.

Tuck Jumps:

    Hold your arms out in front of you parallel to the ground. Use them for balance. Jump up and bring your knees to your chest with your back as straight as possible. Rebound into the next jump immediately. Do ten or twenty jumps.

Hop Sprint:

    Hop forward with both feet together over and over again. As with all tennis jumps rebound into the next jump as soon as possible.

Jumping Rope:

    This is a great exercise that has been used for centuries. Work at it until you can jump pretty fast.

Running:

    This is the basic exercise for all sports. There are three main gaits. If you are running as a rate that can be kept up indefinite then you are jogging. If you are moving at a rate that you could not keep up for ten or twelve minutes and at least one foot is always in contact with the ground then you are running. If you are moving as fast as possible and you are not always in contact with the ground then you are sprinting. Jogging is a good warm up. Running and sprinting are best for tennis training.

Side Steps:

Side Steps are done with the hips parallel to the direction of travel. Spread your feet a little more than shoulder width apart. Bring your feet together by moving your trailing foot towards the other foot. Then step sideways on your leading foot. Do this over and over again and then reverse directions without turning. Do not turn your hips towards the direction of travel in order to get their quicker. Keep your hips parallel to the direction of travel and they will get stronger.

Grapevines:

This classic aerobic exercise it ideal for tennis players. It is similar to a side step. Keep our hips parallel to the direction of travel. If you are moving to the right then bring your left foot in front of your right and reach as far to the right as possible. Then, side step to the right as far as possible. Next, move our left foot behind your right foot as far as possible. Left in front, left behind, left in front, left behind... Repeat going the opposite direction with right in front, right behind... You cannot build up your ability to change direction with side steps and grapevines unless you are strict about keeping your hips parallel to the direction of travel.

Other Great Exercises:

Planks, push-ups and good old fashion jumping jacks are excellent tennis exercises.

Interval Training

High or Medium Intensity Interval Training is a champion maker. There are several ways to do this. The bottom line is to max out (High Intensity) or accelerate (Medium Intensity) your pulse rate. Then, let your pulse rate drop. Max out (High Intensity) or accelerate (Medium Intensity) your pulse rate. Then, let your pulse rate drop. Repeat until you are awesome. The exact exercise that you use to do this is not as relevant as your pulse rate.

You can sprint (High Intensity), run (Medium Intensity), row, ride a bike or use any other method to achieve your goal. Many players like to mix it up to keep from getting bored. The Champions Workout puts many of these classic exercises together in an Interval Training format. Try it.

Champions Workout

The key is to find your max pulse rate. Take 220 and subtract your age. This is your max pulse rate. This is the rate at which you are gasping for breath. Your goal is to put these exercises together so that you exercise at your max pulse rate for 12 to 15 min. You are going to move across the court, do an exercise, move across the court, do an exercise, move etc. ...

Here is an example. After you warm up and stretch, sprint across the court and back from doubles sideline to doubles side line twice. Touch the line each time. As soon as you finish this do 20 squat jumps. Take a ten second break. Next, side step across and back twice, as soon as you finish do 10 pushups. Take a 20 second break and then grapevine across and back twice. Then try 20 lateral jumps. Next hop sprint across and back twice followed by 20 jumping jacks. At this point you should be gasping for breath. Keep up this type of alternate movement and exercises for 12 to 15 min. Stretch again. If you were to do this sort of thing twice a week, mix in two or three jogging sessions of 3 miles each and do at least one wind sprint session a week of at least 8 fifty to one hundred yard sprints, then you would be getting in championship shape. A slow aerobic burn will not cut it if you are training to face tough competition. You need to max out your heart rate for 12 - 15 min, at least three times a week. This is by no means a complete list of the type of exercises that can be effective. The bottom line is your pulse rate. At least 90-95 % of max for 12 to 15 min is what is needed to get you tournament tough. Make sure that your doctor has cleared you for strenuous exercise. Ten to twenty five percent of the time that you spend developing your tennis game should be some type of physical development. Think like a marine. Train as if they were shooting at you.

One Rep - Low Impact Strength Training.

The problem that some people have with weights is that you are stressing your cartilage, ligaments and tendons. It may take a long time to recover if you lift weights in the classic manner. One solution that works for all age groups is to bring a weight half way down and then hold it until you can hold it no more. This will increase your strength but won't take as long to recover from as typical weight lifting. You are increasing your strength but you are not grinding away at the cartilage in your joints to do so. A great leg exercise is to squat until your knee is at a 90 degree angle and then hold it for 60 seconds. Six or seven of these will really boost your leg strength without grinding away at your knees.

A grip exerciser can be used in the same way. Just hold it closed for 2 or 3 minutes and then switch hands and repeat. Do 15 or 20 of these with each hand to improve hand strength without stressing your wrist. This is called "One Rep" Always use at least one spotter when doing a One Rep workout. A great way to do this is to rotate so that the spotter(s) lifts while you spot.

The most basic one rep exercise is the plank. The plank was invented because traditional sit-ups would stretch tendons and ligaments that are better left as short as possible. One Rep is just an extension of this concept to all exercises where heavy weights are being used. Get one or two good spotters and try it. You will tire out your muscles and still not be too sore to recover. If you lift weights in a traditional manner it might take 3 or 4 days before the inflammation is low enough to play tennis at 100%.

Strength is important.  Strength at the price of inflammation is not a good bargain.  One Rep has the lowest chance of causing inflammation.

The effect on your cartilage is even worse. The way that my famous orthopedic guy explained it to me was that your cartilage is like the rubber on a tire. You wear away at it your entire life. When you wear all the way through then you retire from sports.

Basically, if you live long enough your joints will be bone on bone. One Rep will not contribute to this decline. One rep will not grind away at your rubber. Save what cartilage you have for open competition. Your typical weight room is a temple to BFMI.

Combine Practice, Training, & Rest:

You must develop a plan to prepare for each match or tournament.  Here is an example preparation schedule to prepare a typical NCAA player for a match on Saturday.  It begins with the end of a match on the previous Saturday.

Saturday:  Shower, eat, rest (3 hours)

Run 3 miles, Stretch, Champion's workout, one rep workout (total 3 hours)

 Sunday Rest, Warm Up, Stretch. No strenuous physical activity of any kind. (0 hours)

Monday Warm up, stretch, Champion's workout or any HIIT workout (15 min), 2 hours of cooperative practice on the wall, with a partner, or with a coach feeding balls. Use strokes that you can hit all day without stressing your body. Do not force your partner into the defensive mode. Run for 2 or 3 miles. (3 hours total)

Tuesday: Morning workout: warm up, stretch, Champion's workout or any HIIT, Stretch, Hoddle drill for 150 serves, stretch, 1 hour of cooperative and 1 hour of competitive practice. (2.5-3 hours total) Afternoon workout: warm up, stretch, two doubles and two singles practice sets, one rep workout. (2.5-3 hours total)

Wednesday: Rest, Warm Up, Stretch. No strenuous physical activity of any kind. (0 hours)

Thursday: 1000 shot drop hit, 150 count hoodie drill, 3 sets against Wally, and 1 hour of competitive practice. Champions workout or any HIIT workout. (3 – 3.5 hours total)

Friday: 150 count hoodie drill, at least 1 hours of any kind of competitive practice or coach fed drills, at least 2 hours of match play. (3 – 3.5 hours total)

Saturday: Warm up and kick butt!!

Great opponents are defeated by great preparation.

Chapter 20

# Understand the Continental Grip

Use the thumb as the main reference point for this grip. Do not use the 'Base Knuckle" as the main reference point. THIS IS THE MOST IMPORTANT GRIP IN TENNIS. No great players are without this grip. Only topspin ground strokes are hit with a different grip.

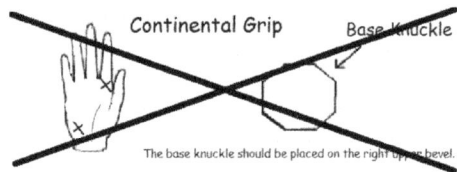

The base knuckle should be placed on the right upper bevel.

This is the way that the Continental Grip is taught. The base knuckle is not the most important reference point for this grip. It is most important to get the thumb in the correct place. The thumb should go straight down to form the correct grip. If you use the base knuckle as your reference point then the grip may or may not get the thumb in the correct place depending on the size of the handle and how thick your grip tape is.

The thumb is the most important reference point for this grip.

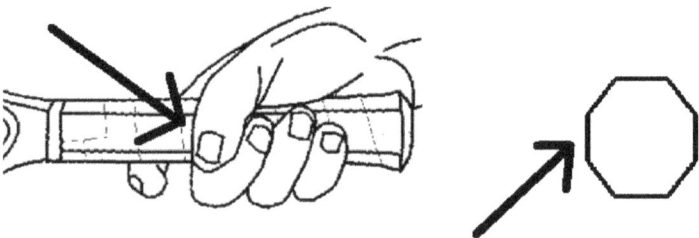

The thumb should go straight down the left side panel of the handle.

If you use the thumb as your reference point then you will have a good grip even if the base knuckle is between bevels or not exactly on the recommended bevel. The thumb is the key. There are more muscles that move the thumb than any other digit. The thumb has a leverage advantage because it is a second class lever and is shorter than most fingers. Let's get the thumb in the right place. Use this grip for every stroke except topspin ground strokes.

Chapter 21

Footwork Goals.

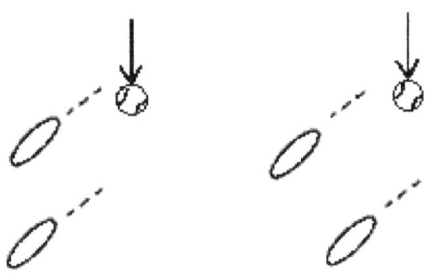

The diagram shows the closed stance and the semi-closed stance. Both can leverage the ball between the shoulders and allow a linear weight shift into the contact point. They are both good hitting stances. The semi-closed stance is a better choice for a two handed shot. There is much debate about which one is better for a one handed forehand. That debate is a red herring. They are both acceptable. If you are using one of these stances then which one you prefer is an irrelevant detail. There is too much discussion about irrelevant details.

The most often over looked aspect of great tennis is foot work. It is real simple. You must get into an acceptable hitting stance that does not cramp you with the ball too close or cause you to reach too far to hit the ball. Left right contact alignment is critical to a good shot. You should try to line up the contact point as soon as possible.

If possible, you need to plant both feet and bend both knees before the power stroke. It is acceptable to come up on the ball of your trailing foot. You cannot shift your weight onto a front foot that is not planted. A great shot can be hit if you are still moving, if you get good alignment at impact. Comfortable contact alignment allows for a linear weight shift into the ball. It will also allow for the ball to be leveraged by the chest muscles. Proper contact alignment is the goal of all footwork.

The impact should take place between the shoulders and not too close or too far away. Do not over-reach or cramp your shots. This footwork goal should be taught at all levels.

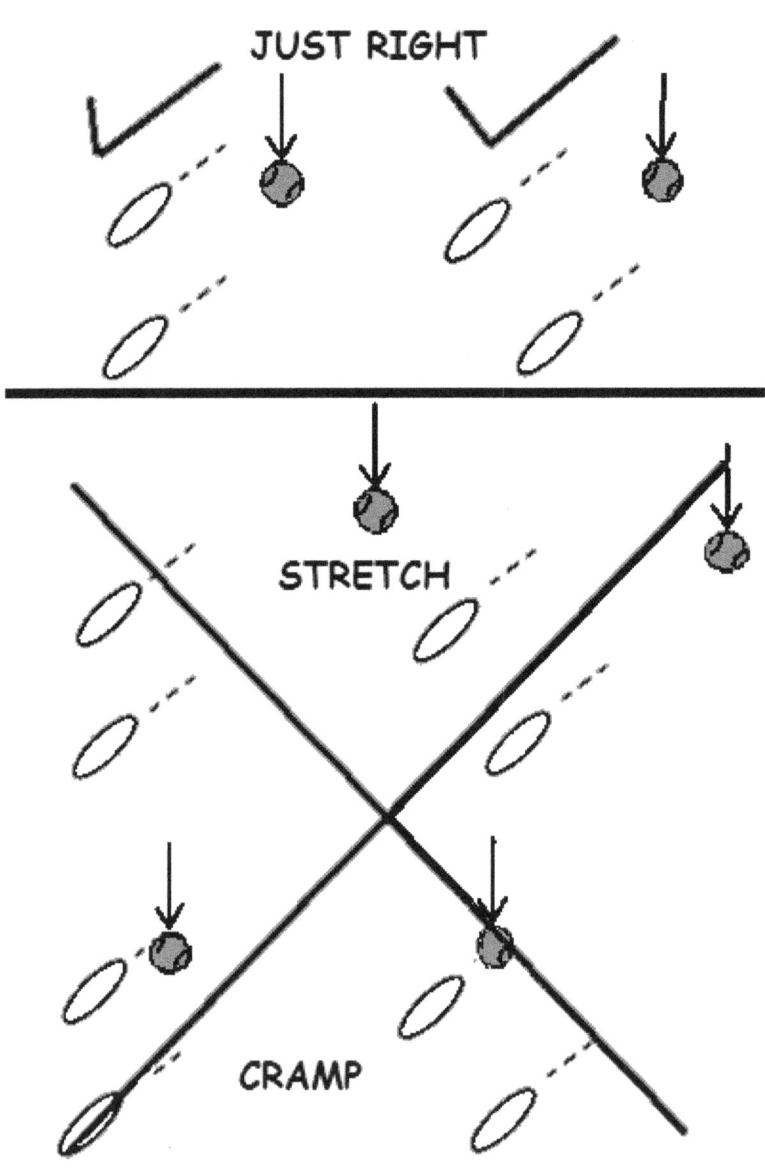

The open stance will never be used to produce a world class offensive shot. If you are in the open stance then you are in the defensive mode.

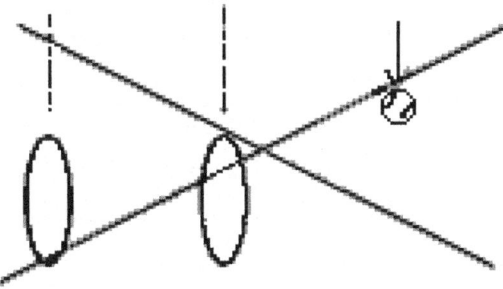

You cannot leverage the ball between your hips and shoulders or shift your weight into a shot if you use the open stance. Rotating the upper body is a poor substitute for this.

## Conclusion

Most 5.0 players spend less time in lessons and more time preparing with workouts and practice. There are pros who are good at preparing a 5.0 or above player. These pros are more physical and tactical in their approach than most instructors and typically are very good at what they do. Most teaching pros will deal with one of these four elements in each lesson; backswing, follow through, foot work, bending the knees. When they fix all of these four things they often go into greater and greater detail about the exact form of each shot. If you are bending your knees, planting your front foot, getting your racket back, planning and observing a good impact configuration, and following through then there is limited value in concentration on the less important details of style. Sadly most modern players and instructors ignore targeting skills. Many of today's players, even on the pro tour have beautiful shots that too often land on the service line. Of course, you need to learn how to produce a good looking, efficient, proper stroke. However, you do not need to keep learning this over and over again.

If you are a player who is taking the time to become really great at tennis then your best choice for a teaching pro is one who challenges you physically. The ideal choice would a pro who treats the racket like an exercise machine and gives you a great physical workout on court as you hit a lot of balls. The best teaching pros for an elite player are the ones who give you just enough time to set up into a good hitting stance.

Evaluate your teaching pros and coaches based on the magic number. You need, "a little less talk and a lot more action." You should also film yourself and watch yourself on a regular basis. When you see the video of your shots in slow motion do not leave out checking to see that you are following the ball all the way to impact and holding your focus long enough to read the details with your peripheral vision.

Use every shot to practice your targeting and impact feedback system. Every time that you see a person hit a tennis ball you should take the 1/75 of a second to hold your focus on the impact point and read every impact detail. You will soon see that the better players use the impact configurations outlined in this book. Use the Champion's pattern even if you can beat a player with BFMI. You will still beat them quickly and you need to make this your normal game.

Instead of Brute Force Mass Ignorance, try Brute Force Mass Intelligence. You need great strokes, a visual targeting and cybernetic feedback system, patterned strategic play, great physical conditioning, mental toughness and the ability to refocus from a distraction. You cannot leave any of these important aspect out of your development or you will have a built in weakness.

There is often a debate in tennis circles about which is better power or consistency. Do not fall into the either/or trap of this mindset. If you build your game around visual skills and discipline you can have a powerful consistent game. "Throw the power" to a spot. Adjust that spot.

Marvin Dent was right. Federer is Betterer. Typically instructors will not use Federer as a model because his strokes do not always look consistently the same. He is lining up and creating each shot as a unique optimum response. His dynamic approach is what needs to be copied.

As tennis players we are bombarded with statistics every time we watch a match. There are useful, but they are not as useful as the one statistic that you need to estimate every time you play or practice. After every point or rally assess how many shots you held your focus on until you noticed every detail of the impact. I like to estimate what my visual discipline percentage is every match. You are the only one who can estimate this. It is possible to ignore the impact even if your face is pointed at the ball as the strings stretch. If you make this informal estimate then I assure you that you will soon realize that when your visual discipline percentage is at 100% for any point, game, set, or match, that is when you are playing your best tennis. A visual discipline percentage at 100% means that you are in the zone. You have formed the tennis trance.

Play smart. Play strong. Do not let anyone beat you unless they can beat your best strong, intelligent, disciplined game. Celebrate victories. Go and conquer the world.

Made in the USA
Las Vegas, NV
08 June 2021